PUBLIC HEALTH IN THE 21ST CENTURY

# PUBLIC HEALTH AND HARM REDUCTION

# PRINCIPLES, PERCEPTIONS AND PROGRAMS

# Public Health in the 21st Century

Additional books in this series can be found on Nova's website under the Series tab.

Additional e-books in this series can be found on Nova's website under the e-book tab.

PUBLIC HEALTH IN THE 21ST CENTURY

# PUBLIC HEALTH AND HARM REDUCTION

## PRINCIPLES, PERCEPTIONS AND PROGRAMS

MEREDITH B. MORRIS
EDITOR

nova publishers
*New York*

## NOTICE TO THE READER



Additional color graphics may be available in the e-book version of this book.

**Library of Congress Cataloging-in-Publication Data**

ISBN: 978-1-63482-159-9
Library of Congress Control Number: 2015931778

*Published by Nova Science Publishers, Inc. † New York*

# CONTENTS

**Preface** **vii**

**Chapter 1** Preventing School Shootings: A Public Health Approach to Gun-Related Homicide and Murder-Suicide in Schools **1**
*David N. Miller and Kristin D. Sawka-Miller*

**Chapter 2** Enlarging the Social Definition of Harm to Include Genetics **35**
*Stephen M. Modell, Sharon L. R. Kardia and Toby Citrin*

**Chapter 3** Endocrine Disruptors, Obesity and Public Health: Perspectives on Harm Reduction **47**
*Minelli Salles Alves Fernandes, Melvy Marin Rivero, Marcela Miranda Salles, Denise Rosso Tenório Wanderley Rocha and Alberto Krayyem Arbex*

**Chapter 4** Tobacco Public Health and Harm Reduction: Principles, Perceptions and Programs **63**
*Marcia Erazo, Maria Paz Bertoglia, Juan Guillermo Gormaz, Matías Libuy and Carla Bertossi*

**Chapter 5** Smoking-Related Disengagement Beliefs among Smoking Asthma Patients **83**
*Efrat Neter, Gal Gida and Ella Eliya*

**Chapter 6** Public Health and Waste Management: Promoting Harm Reduction Through Concerted Efforts **93**
*Vitalis Chukwuemeka Echebiri BMLS, AIMLS, MPH*

**Chapter 7** Harm Reduction for People Who Inject Drugs through Point of Care CD4/Viral Load Testing in Kenya **117**
*Kennedy Kinyua, Eva Muluve, Paul Macharia and Helgar Musyoki*

**Chapter 8** Medication Assisted Therapy Integrating Mobile Phone Technologies **125**
*Paul Macharia, Eva Muluve and Helgar Musyoki*

**Index** **135**

# PREFACE

Public health is a part of the health system whose researchers' have tried to maintain its relevance over the years amidst unstable global conditions. Maintaining its tripartite objective of promoting health, preventing diseases and prolonging life is a major hurdle especially as these functions have to depend on the combined efforts of society. This book focuses on principles, perceptions and programs of public health. Some of the topics discussed in this book include school shootings, waste management and public health, and tobacco use.

Chapter 1 - School shootings have received substantial media attention in recent years, largely due to the increased incidents of gun violence in schools and the number of casualties and deaths that have occurred as a result. These acts of gun violence have frequently resulted in the deaths of perpetrators as well as victims and include incidents of homicide, suicide, and murder-suicide. Consequently, school personnel, parents, law enforcement, and policy makers have become increasingly concerned about school shootings and how to most effectively prevent them. The purpose of this chapter is to describe a public health approach to school shootings, with a particular emphasis on preventing homicide and murder-suicide in schools. Both school–based and community–based approaches for preventing school shootings are reviewed, including restricting access to guns among young people, identifying potentially homicidal and suicidal youth through threat and risk assessments, and effective crisis response and intervention.

Chapter 2 - Harm can be both physical and social, a function of the health-related ethos that society adopts. Ecological models clarify that harm can result from acts of commission and omission occurring at the genetic, not just gross, level. In this commentary we present examples of harm reduction from the public health genetics literature that touch on positive actions which may be taken to promote primary, secondary, and tertiary disease prevention. The avoidance of neural tube defects through cereal fortification, dietary prevention of newborn metabolic defects, and genetic testing to avoid pernicious spread of hereditary breast and ovarian cancer occupy these categories of harm reduction, each touching on starkly visible harms that could take place without proper public health efforts. Neighborhoods in low income areas in multiple countries present challenging conditions. Poor nutritional food availability and the possibility of environmental contaminants, lead being a widespread example, require attention to avoid exposure in one generation resulting in harm to the next. Genetic research has uncovered the epigenetic mechanisms behind the gene-environment interactions that may result. The solutions are both biological and social, with community resources playing a part. The unique contribution of public health genetics to the field of harm reduction is the awareness it has raised of the distinction between genotypic and phenotypic prevention, especially in the realm of prenatal genetic testing. This distinction has impacted the United States more so than other countries in terms of the range of services offered by public health authorities, and has helped to avoid labeling and stigmatization that might otherwise occur through the prevention of human characteristics. An educated public health workforce can maximize the benefits of genetic policies for physical harm reduction while minimizing the use of interventions that could otherwise result in social harm.

Chapter 3 - Endocrine-disrupting Chemicals (EDCs) are exogenous chemicals that interfere with the metabolism and action of various hormones and intracellular signaling. The interference in the differentiation of adipocytes and weight homeostasis are key actions of EDCs, which could possibly be associated with obesity. EDCs may also have effects during intrauterine development, contributing to increase an individual's weight in adulthood. Obesity is a pandemic nowadays, increasing especially among children, and also in developing countries. It is a chronic inflammatory multifactorial disease. Current studies suggest a possible association with pre or postnatal exposure to endocrine disruptors. These 'obesogenic' disruptors are found in food packaging, cosmetics, industrial waste, organochlorine pesticides and fuels. The most common contaminants are Bisphenol A (BPA), phthalates, phytoestrogens, dioxine and DDT. Despite the correlation between increased body mass and adipogenesis by the action of EDCs, their molecular mechanisms remain poorly understood. These substances affect the endocrine function by stimulating PPARy receptors or acting as antiandrogens -

aromatase inhibitors, resulting in increased lipogenesis. Those receptors are associated the differentiation, activation and maturation of adipocytes in fat synthesis in cells. They can also act on nuclear receptors and on the nervous system. Several factors such as age and length of exposure can influence the effect of EDCs, but the dose-response relationship remains unclear. The goal of this chapter is to develop a critical review of the literature on the influence of environmental contaminants in the development of adiposity.

Chapter 4 - Tobacco consumption is a worldwide epidemic that causes illness and mortality at all ages, sexes and countries. In order to protect population of damages of active and passive smoking, the World Health Organization (WHO), in accordance to the principles of the Charter of United Nations that promotes the right of people to enjoy the highest attainable standard of health without distinction of race, religion, and political belief, economic or social condition, developed a framework for tobacco control. The WHO Framework Convention on Tobacco Control (FCTC) is an international treaty that provides evidence-based recommendations for health promotion and tobacco control. Among the strategies that have been implemented worldwide to curve the epidemic of tobacco smoking are: smoking ban in public places, package labelling, to remove vending machines, health promotion for school-children and at workplaces, increase taxes, tobacco cessation programs, among others. Complete smoking ban in public places is a successful policy; several studies in different countries have shown a reduction in myocardial infarction after few months of the policy implementation. Other strategies have been less implemented and not fully evaluated. Limited political commitment and limited human capital expertise are examples of perceived barriers that were identified by countries to implement in a proper manner the FCTC. An increase in country capacity building and technical cooperation between countries are priorities to secure worldwide implementation of FCTC.

Chapter 5 - *Background:* Though smoking accelerates asthma, smoking is actually more common among asthmatics. A possible explanation for this discrepancy is that asthmatics use more techniques such as disengagement beliefs to reduce the dissonance between their knowledge on the deleterious effects of smoking and their behavior. Disengagement beliefs are beliefs that minimize the behavior and are generated in order to explain / justify non-congruent behaviors

*Methods:* Participants (n=199, 94 asmathics and 105 non-asthmatics filled out a self-reported on-line questionnaire measuring disengagement beliefs and the Brief Illness Perception Questionnaire. Disengagement beliefs were predicted by two independent variables: Asthma and smoking status.

*Results:* Smokers used significantly more smoking-related disengagement beliefs than non smokers. An interaction between smoking and asthma status was significant so that asthmatic smokers held significantly more smoking-related disengagement beliefs than non-asthmatic smokers and all other combinations. Additionally, asthmatic smokers reported significantly less control over their illness and a significantly poorer understanding of their disease than non-smoking asthmatics. In contrast to the hypothesis, asthmatic smokers reported experiencing more symptoms and more consequences to their illness than non-smoking asthmatics.

*Conclusion:* Increased use of smoking-related disengagement beliefs among asthmatic smokers has limited impact, as indicated in the higher level of perceived consequences and reported symptoms of the illness among them, compared to non-smoking asthmatics. Disengagement beliefs provide an explanation for the seeming contradiction between smoking and asthma, and may provide clues for future interventions.

Chapter 6 - This chapter examines the risk posed by the increasing waste generation all over the world, and proposes harm reduction through global concerted efforts. Industrial revolution and sustained urban growth have resulted in massive generation of various kinds of wastes. Sanitary conditions have therefore continued to worsen, leading to population harm and painful reduction in the overall quality of life due to breeding of diseases and outbreaks. Most often, the unexpected rise in the number of disease cases overwhelms the available health facilities leading to preventable deaths. Although legislations to manage wastes abound in various countries, the rate of generation outweighs the capacity to manage these wastes. Regrettably, some countries generate very toxic wastes which are illegally transported to unsuspecting countries for disposal, not minding the harm these will cause the population in those countries. This action undermines the global campaign for good health for all, and therefore calls for global commitment toward a better and safer waste management mechanism geared toward promoting cleaner and healthier environment with concomitant harm reduction to the global population.

Chapter 7 - Global HIV/AIDS disease among people who inject drugs is significant and expanding. Unsafe injecting drug use has resulted in the rapid spread of HIV among drug user networks in countries throughout the world. In Kenya, injecting drug use (IDU) is an emerging problem which needs urgent attention because of its close association with the rapid spread of HIV which can potentiate local HIV epidemics.

Injecting drug users don't access health care services due to socio-economic factors like absence of empathy, listening, shaming, discrimination, flexibility, lack of disclosure and the cost of health care.

Focused and evidence-based approaches are needed to combat IDU-related HIV in Kenya. In resource-constrained settings like Kenya, it is difficult to do viral load and CD4 cell measurements to start treatment but instead rely on clinical staging. But Studies have shown WHO HIV staging misses many with low CD4.

Researchers have therefore been working to make viral load and CD4 cell testing machines which are cheaper, more accessible and easier to use.

Point of care viral load and CD4 machines could then be introduced into the most remote settings in Kenya to help put more people onto care on the basis of viral load and CD4 counts rather than staging. The new tests would also facilitate the delivery of ART in decentralized settings and possibly improve retention into ART programmes, by speeding the time it takes between when a person gets tested and when he or she goes onto ART.

Chapter 8 - Accurate harm reduction information is needed if clients are to make informed choices, this can be achieved by strategically improving and availing this information. There are a number of available harm-reduction strategies that are promising have been very successful. The importance of individualizing harm reduction intervention to accommodate the preferences and needs of a targeted person or population cannot be over emphasized. A good harm reduction effort will seek to meet the individual where he or she is at and assist that person in the direction of positive behavior change.

Information and communication technologies could increase access by providing individualized up-to-date harm reduction information to promote health, reduce harm, and support client access to care. Cheaper, efficient and reliable mobile phones avail technological opportunities to offer secure and confidential access to harm reduction information. This could include developing mobile phone applications that would ensure easy access to up-to-date information thus enhancing client literacy.

In: Public Health and Harm Reduction
Editor: Meredith B. Morris
ISBN: 978-1-63482-159-9


*Chapter 1*

# Preventing School Shootings: A Public Health Approach to Gun-Related Homicide and Murder-Suicide in Schools

***David N. Miller[1,*] and Kristin D. Sawka-Miller[2]***
[1]University at Albany, State University of New York, NY, US
[2]Siena College, Loudonville, NY, US

## Abstract

School shootings have received substantial media attention in recent years, largely due to the increased incidents of gun violence in schools and the number of casualties and deaths that have occurred as a result. These acts of gun violence have frequently resulted in the deaths of perpetrators as well as victims and include incidents of homicide, suicide, and murder-suicide. Consequently, school personnel, parents, law enforcement, and policy makers have become increasingly concerned about school shootings and how to most effectively prevent them. The purpose of this chapter is to describe a public health approach to school shootings, with a particular emphasis on preventing homicide and murder-suicide in schools. Both school–based and community–based approaches for preventing school shootings are reviewed, including restricting access to guns among young people, identifying potentially

* Corresponding author: David N. Miller. E-mail: dmiller@albany.edu.

homicidal and suicidal youth through threat and risk assessments, and effective crisis response and intervention.

## INTRODUCTION

School shootings are horrific and tragic events that have devastating effects on students, schools, and communities. Although far more common in the United States than in other nations, school shootings are a global phenomenon, having occurred in at least 23 countries and in each of the world's continents (Bondü, Scheithauer, Leuschner, and Cornell, 2013). Böckler and his colleagues (2013 a,b) reported that there were 120 instances of school shootings between 1925 and 2011, with 76 of them (63.3%) occurring in the US. There has been a notable increase in school shootings in the last few decades (Böckler et al., 2013 a,b), accompanied by a correspondingly larger number of individuals wounded and killed.

The most lethal cases of school shootings, such as the incidents at Columbine High School in 1999 and Sandy Hook Elementary School in 2012, have received widespread media attention and resulted in greater public fear and uncertainty about the safety of schools (Bondü et al., 2013; Borum, Cornell, Modzeleski, and Jimerson, 2010). This has occurred despite the extreme rarity of school shootings, as well as clear evidence that schools are among the safest places for children and youth to be (Jimerson, Hart, and Renshaw, 2012). School shootings are such inherently disturbing events, however, that they often generate inflated perceptions of danger and vulnerability (Cornell, 2006). Highly publicized news media reports, which often speculate about emerging and bogus "trends" based on highly unusual cases, further exacerbate public fears and anxieties (Borum et al., 2010). Consequently, many well-intentioned but ineffective efforts to make schools safer have proliferated, often predicated on "unrealistic appraisals of risk and misunderstanding about the nature of the actual threat" (Borum et al., 2010, p. 27).

In the United States, although many Americans likely view school shootings as a relatively recent development, this is unfortunately not the case. The first known school shooting in the US occurred in Pennsylvania in 1764 and involved the murder of a teacher and several students by Native American warriors in the aftermath of the French and Indian War. Since that initial incident, newspaper accounts indicate that multiple school shootings have occurred in US schools, colleges, and universities during every decade since the 1850s. Notable increases in school shootings began in the late twentieth century, and historically higher rates have continued into the twenty–first century.

Unfortunately, due to a variety of methodological problems and limitations, accurately predicting and effectively preventing school shootings presents an enormous challenge to school personnel, law enforcement, parents, and policy makers (Borum et al., 2010; Cornell and Williams, 2012). One major methodological and conceptual problem is the lack of a consistent definition of the phenomenon (Bondü et al., 2013). Although there is general agreement that school shootings can be defined as "offenses by a present or former student who purposely chooses his or her school as the site to carry out an attempt to kill one or more persons" (Bondü et al., 2013, p. 343), there is no consensus on the details of that definition. For example, the definition might include any attempt to kill one or more individuals, regardless of the outcome, or it might be limited to those cases in which one or more individuals are actually killed (Bondü et al., 2013).

Questions have also been raised regarding whether prior planning is required and whether a firearm must be used for an incident to be classified as a school shooting. Because some perpetrators have used weapons other than firearms (e.g., the most deadly school massacre in US history occurred in 1927 and involved the bombing of a school in Bath Township, Michigan by a disgruntled school board member), many alternatives to the phrase "school shootings" have been suggested, including "school rampage," "lethal school violence," "targeted violence in schools," and "homicidal violence in schools" (Bondü et al., 2013, p. 344). Most of these terms, however, have the converse problem of being too broad by not sufficiently differentiating school shootings from other acts of lethal violence in schools. Consequently, these variations in definition not only affect the selection of cases for study but also lead to differing calculations of their frequency, hindering comparisons across studies (Bondü et al., 2013).

Perhaps the most significant challenge in better predicting school shootings, however, is their low frequency or base rate (Mulvey and Cauffman, 2001). Although a low base rate for such horrific and tragic events is of course highly desirable, it does make accurate prediction of such incidents extremely difficult. For example, over the course of a 10–year period the United States averaged 21 student homicide fatalities per year. Although the violent deaths of 21 students annually is highly troubling, with approximately 125,000 schools in the US the average school can expect the homicidal death of a student about once every 6,000 years (Borum et al.,

2010). In another example, Germany has approximately 43,500 schools and experienced 12 school shootings in a 13–year period. The average school in Germany can therefore expect a similar attack once every 40,000 years. Consequently, simply predicting that no student will carry out a school shooting will be accurate more than 99.99% of the time (Bondü et al., 2013). Clearly, there are inherent limits to predicting acts of extreme school violence (Mulvey and Cauffman, 2001), and these limitations are largely due to their low base rate in the population and the associated difficulties resulting from it.

## School Shootings and School–Associated Homicides

An important distinction should be made between school shootings and school–associated homicides. According to the Centers for Disease Control and Prevention (CDC), between 14 and 34 students between the ages of 5 and 18 are killed at or on their way to or from school each year, which represents between 1 and 2% of all homicides in that age group. Most of these school–associated homicides, however, would not be considered school shootings per se. Like other juvenile homicides, most school–associated homicides tend to be gang–related, drug–related, or linked to interpersonal disputes or criminal activities in which the school is simply the site for the attack (Borum et al., 2010). In contrast, school shootings like the ones that occurred at Columbine High School in Colorado and Sandy Hook Elementary School in Connecticut represent a particularly rare subtype of school–associated homicides. The US Secret Service and Department of Education Safe School Initiative referred to these cases as "targeted school–based attacks" because it was important to the perpetrator(s) that the shooting occur at a specific school, unlike those cases in which an intended target just happened to be at the school (Vossekuil, Fein, Reddy, Borum, and Modzeleski, 2002).

## Laws, Initiatives, and Strategies for Preventing School Shootings

Several laws, initiatives, and strategies have been implemented with the goal of increasing school safety, particularly in regards to gun–related violence in schools. Borum and his colleagues (2010) identified several of these developments, including the Gun–Free School Act, zero tolerance policies, persistently dangerous schools, target hardening and security measures, and the use of profiling, risk factors, and warning signs. Each of these strategies is described briefly below.

## Gun–Free School Act

The Gun–Free School Act (GFSA), part of the Improving America's Schools Act, was passed in 1994. The GFSA called for states to enact laws requiring that a student be expelled for a period of not less than one year if the student brings a firearm to school or possesses a firearm at school. The law was passed during a time period in which the rate of violent behavior in schools was near its peak (Dinkes, Cataldi, and Lin–Kelly, 2007). The GFSA was designed to target the possession of firearms in schools, but because the law gave authority to states to pass their own legislation, many states broadened the possible behaviors for which students might be expelled. For example, many states enacted bills that required expulsion not only for firearm possession at school but also for offenses such as selling drugs, making threats, and assaulting teachers. Consequently, the passage of the GFSA is viewed by many as the beginning of the zero–tolerance movement (Borum et al., 2010).

## Zero Tolerance

The term *zero tolerance* refers to "a range of policies that seek to impose severe sanctions – in schools, typically suspension and expulsion – for minor offenses in hopes of preventing more serious ones" (Borum et al., 2010, p. 28). The philosophy underlying zero tolerance is that particular behaviors deemed inappropriate will be dealt with swiftly and consistently, ultimately resulting in greater deterrence (Skiba, Shure, Middelberg, and Baker, 2012). In accordance with this philosophy, school administrators have sometimes overreacted by employing suspension and expulsion for a variety of relatively innocuous behaviors, including the possession of paper or toy guns and over–the–counter medications, such as Advil (American Psychological Association Zero Tolerance Task Force, 2008).

Despite their prevalence, zero tolerance policies have been widely criticized because they have not demonstrated to serve as a deterrent to future occurrences of misbehavior (Borum et al., 2010; Skiba et al., 2012). Longitudinal studies of suspensions resulting from zero tolerance policies have consistently found high rates of repeat offending following out–of–school suspensions (Skiba et al., 2012). For example, Raffaele–Mendez (2003) found that the best predictor of a middle school student's number of out–of–school suspensions was the number of out–of–school suspensions the student received in late elementary school (i.e., fourth or fifth grade), even after controlling for variables such as student socio–economic status, special education status, racial categorization, academic achievement, and teacher ratings of student behavior. In addition, the legality of zero tolerance policies has been questioned, they have been criticized as being contrary to the principles of healthy child and adolescent development, and they have raised serious concerns about the frequency of their racially disproportionate application (Borum et al., 2010; Skiba et al., 2012).

## Persistently Dangerous Schools

A section of the Elementary and Secondary Education Act of 1965 (as amended by the No Child Left Behind Act of 2001) required that states develop policies to give students more choice in regards to the school they are attending if the one they are currently attending presents safety problems. More specifically, students were permitted to attend a "safe school" of their choice within their school district if the student attended a "persistently dangerous school" or became a victim of a violent crime (as defined by the state) while in school or on school grounds. Referred to as the Unsafe School Choice Option, this provision did not provide criteria for how states should define a persistently dangerous school or a time frame for students to transfer to a safe school (Mayer and Leone, 2007).

The persistently dangerous school initiative has been criticized on a number of levels. For example, a large majority of states chose to use the number of student suspensions and expulsions as the criterion for designating schools as being "persistently dangerous." Although this metric makes use of readily available data, the validity of this approach is unclear. Moreover, some state officials did not act on the persistently dangerous schools initiative and relatively few schools have been designated as being "persistently dangerous," leading many observers to the conclusion that they dramatically underestimate the actual number of dangerous schools. It has been suggested that school officials may underestimate or underreport incidents of violence in schools in order to avoid being labeled as persistently dangerous (Borum et al., 2010; Mayer and Leone, 2007).

## Target Hardening and Security Measures

The term *target hardening* refers to procedures for preventing crimes or limiting the opportunity for crimes to be committed by creating protective barriers. Schools in the US have been engaged in target hardening and other security measures for several decades (Borum et al., 2010). Currently, schools make use of a variety of security measures, including requesting visitors to sign in (93%), placing school staff in hallways (90%), locking school entranceways and/or exit doors during the school day (54%), and searching school lockers (53%; Dinkes, Cataldi, and Lin–Kelly, 2007).

More schools are also using cameras for surveillance purposes, including stationary analog cameras and, more recently, digital cameras that can pan across particular areas and be monitored by multiple observers (Grant, 2003). Unfortunately, the effects of security cameras on behavior in schools have not been studied extensively (Borum et al., 2010) and studies of camera surveillance in other settings (e.g., closed circuit television) have reported mixed results (e.g., Gill and Sprigs, 2005; Welsh and Farrington, 2002, 2004). Some research has found that conspicuously placed security cameras may reduce unruly public behavior (Priks, 2008) and increase prosocial behavior (van Rompay, Vonk, and Fransen, 2009), suggesting that an individual's level of awareness of the presence of a camera may influence its effects (Borum et al., 2010). Unfortunately, there is no current evidence that surveillance cameras, including those conspicuously posted, will deter school shooters.

In the wake of school shootings, there has been an increased emphasis within many schools on requiring students and staff to wear badges or picture ID in order to enter the school, and to have controlled access to schools monitored by school personnel. Metal detectors, designed to detect any firearms students may possess, have also been used with increasing frequency in schools, and some schools have resorted to hiring police and security guards. To date, however, there is little empirical research available evaluating these practices (Borum et al., 2010) and what little research has occurred has sometimes reported negative outcomes. For example, as schools increase their reliance on physical means to deter violence (i.e., metal detectors, surveillance cameras, locked doors), there is often a concomitant increase in student fear and disorder (Bachman, Randolph, and Brown, 2011; Mayer, 2010; Mayer and

Leone, 1999; Perumean-Chaney and Sutton, 2013). Similarly, students report feeling less safe when there is heavy reliance on security personnel (Bachman et al., 2011; Mayer, 2010), particularly in the absence of a positive school climate, and the presence of school security officers has been associated with more arrests for disorderly conduct (Theriot, 2009).

The combined findings suggest that criminalizing student behavior and creating arguably unwelcoming, "prison-like" schools may actually increase the likelihood of school violence. Moreover, the presence of any of these security measures does not necessarily mean that school shootings will be more effectively prevented. For example, both surveillance cameras and security guards were present but did not prevent the school shootings at Columbine High School in Colorado or at Red Lake High School in Minnesota. As Langman (2009 a,b) notes, such security measures will have much less impact if individuals are highly motivated to kill, have access to firearms, and are actively suicidal (as was the case with the Columbine and Red Lake school shooters).

## Profiling, Risk Factors, and Warnings Signs

*Profiling* refers to the practice, made popular by the FBI and law enforcement, of developing particular "profiles" of criminals based on demographic and other data–based variables (Owen, 2004).In the aftermath of extensive media coverage of the school shootings at Columbine High School in April of 1999, some authorities identified what they believed to be certain similarities across multiple cases and suggested that there might be a profile of the "typical" school shooter (Band and Harpold, 1999; McGee and DeBernardo, 1999).

There is clear and compelling evidence, however, indicating that efforts to profile students is an inherently flawed process (Heilbrun, Dvoskin, and Heilbrun, 2009). For example, the US Secret Service and the US Department of Education conducted a systematic review of targeted school shootings and found there was no accurate or useful demographic or social profile of school shooters (Fein et al., 2002; Vossekuil et al., 2002). Subsequent research has continued to support the conclusion that there is no practical and useful profile of a "typical" school shooter (American Psychological Association, 2013; Heilbrun et al., 2009). Although the US Secret Service and Department of Education did find some common characteristics associated with school shooters (e.g., being male; having a history of peer mistreatment and bullying;

demonstrating a preoccupation with violent video games and fantasies), these characteristics are extremely limited in their utility (Fein et al., 2002). Moreover, the use of profiling has been criticized because of its potential for inaccurately and unfairly labeling particular students as being dangerous and consequently restricting their civil liberties (Sewell and Mendelsohn, 2000).

There are similar problems associated with examining risk factors and warning signs associated with school shootings. Risk factors refer to variables that may predispose an individual to certain behaviors and are typically long–standing, often unchangeable, and have a distant temporal relationship to the behavior of interest. In contrast, warning signs tend to be more dynamic and indicate the more immediate possibility of a crisis. In regards to risk factors, there are significant challenges in making predictions about school behavior based on them even when very large samples are used. For example, Furlong and colleagues (2001, 2004) used data from the Youth Risk Behavior Surveillance Survey (one of their studies included more than 40,000 students) to predict self–reported weapon carrying in school. Although the researchers were able to identify a statistically significant, moderate correlation between weapon carrying and the nine strongest predictors, they concluded that these predictors were inadequate and impractical at the individual student level, largely because even the most accurate prediction would falsely identify a large number of students as being weapon carriers (i.e., there would be a high number of "false positives"). These researchers also found that the most frequent weapon carriers in schools were much more likely to have zero school risk factors than to have many of them (Furlong et al., 2001).

Similar challenges exist for using warning signs to accurately identify students at risk for more general behavior problems, such as getting into fights or exhibiting anger (American Psychological Association, 1999; Borum et al., 2010; Dwyer, Osher, and Warger, 1998). Although some warning sign checklists that have been developed explicitly state that the checklist neither constitutes a profile nor predicts violent behavior (e.g., Dwyer et al., 1998), it is not clear whether these cautions are attended to or heeded in practice (Sewell and Mendelsohn, 2000).

In sum, the use of profiling has not received empirical support for identifying potential school shooters or in predicting which students are most likely to become school shooters (American Psychological Association, 2013; Borum et al., 2010). In fact, one of the conclusions made by the FBI report was that profiling was not an appropriate method for preventing school shootings, and that "trying to draw up a catalogue or 'checklist' of warning signs to detect a potential school shooter can be shortsighted, even dangerous.

Such lists, publicized by the media, can end up unfairly labeling many nonviolent students as potentially dangerous" (O'Toole, 2000, p. 2).

## LEAKAGE

The Safe Schools Initiative, a joint study conducted by the US Secret Service and the US Department of Education, examined detailed case studies of 37 targeted school attacks involving 41 perpetrators over a 25 year period (Vossekuil et al., 2002). These investigators found that all the attackers were male and that guns were nearly always the weapon of choice used in the attacks. Moreover, the attacks were found to be rarely, if ever, impulsive. The majority of school shooters were found to have made a plan at least two days prior to the incident; in some cases, the planning had gone on for up to a year (Vossekuil et al., 2002).

Perhaps the most salient finding from this analysis, however, and the one with arguably the greatest practical value, was that in three–quarters of the incidents the perpetrators told someone about their interest and plans in mounting an attack at the school. Perpetrators typically informed friends or other peers, and in more than half the cases multiple people knew about the attacks before their occurrence, although they rarely communicated a threat directly to the target of the attack (Vossekuil et al., 2002).

The finding that school shooters typically communicated their intentions in some way to others prior to their attacks – a practice referred to by the FBI as "leakage" – raised the possibility that school shootings "could conceivably be prevented by investigating situations in which a student was known to make a threat of violence, communicate intent, or otherwise engage in behavior suggesting plans or preparations for a school–based attack" (Borum et al., 2010, p. 31). This process, known as threat assessment, is discussed in greater detail later in this chapter.

## SUICIDAL BEHAVIOR, MURDER–SUICIDE, AND SCHOOL SHOOTERS

Although suicide and violence prevention efforts have generally occurred in relative isolation from each other (Lubell and Vetter, 2006), there is increasing evidence suggesting that self–directed violence and interpersonal violence frequently overlap (Joiner, 2014; Miller, 2012a; Nickerson and Slater, 2009). Additionally, human beings (as well as other living organisms) appear to have a natural (presumably biological) barrier against within–species killing, and this applies to killing oneself as well as others (Grossman, 1995; Joiner, 2014). In order to overcome this natural barrier, repeated exposure to violence in some form, and eventually habituating to it, appears to be a critical variable in cases of murder as well as suicide (Grossman, 1995; Joiner, 2005, 2014).

The relationship between self–directed violence and interpersonal violence can be seen in the context of school shootings (Miller, 2011; Miller and Mazza, in press; Preti, 2008). For example, the Secret Service and Department of Education study found that 78% of the school shooters they examined exhibited suicidal ideation to a significant degree (Vossekuil et al., 2002). In their list of worldwide school rampage shootings that occurred between 1925 and 2011, Böckler and his colleagues (2013a) found that the perpetrators of school shootings also killed themselves in over one–quarter (26.6%) of the incidents – a rate much higher than murder–suicides that occur in other settings (Joiner, 2014). Moreover, an examination of the six school shooting incidents in the US with the highest number of fatalities indicates that five of them involved the suicide of the perpetrator(s). The one case that was not technically a suicide (the 1966 school shootings that occurred on the campus of the University of Texas at Austin) was, in all likelihood, a case of "suicide by cop" (i.e., a situation in which a suicidal individual intentionally acts in a threatening way toward law enforcement with the goal of provoking a lethal response). Further supporting this contention is the fact that the perpetrator left a suicide note (Joiner, 2014).

School personnel, in particular, may not be sufficiently aware that many incidents of school shootings involve the suicide of the perpetrators as well as the murder of innocent victims (Langman, 2009 a,b, 2013; Vossekuil et al., 2002). In fact, Joiner (2014) has provided compelling evidence that it is suicide – not murder – that is the initial and primary motivation among individuals who commit murder–suicide, and a similar conclusion has been made by researchers studying suicide bombers in the Middle East (Lankford, 2013; Lankford and Hakim, 2011). For example, the two perpetrators in the infamous school shooting incident at Columbine High School (i.e., Eric Harris and Dylan Klebold) were each suicidal. Suicidal ideation was particularly pronounced in Klebold, who had been actively thinking about killing himself for at least two years prior to the school shootings (Cullen, 2009) and whose journals indicated that he expected to be dead by suicide months before the tragedy at Columbine occurred (Joiner, 2014).

Joiner (2014) has also proposed that perpetrators of murder–suicide invariably pervert one of four interpersonal virtues – justice, mercy, duty, and/or heroic glory. Although Joiner (2014) suggests that in most cases of murder–suicide perversions of justice (e.g., in which the perpetrator believes that justice would be served by killing at least one other person in addition to himself/herself) and mercy (e.g., in which the perpetrator believes it would be merciful to kill someone else in addition to himself/herself, such as a suicidal husband who believes it would be "merciful" to kill his spouse as well because she would be "better off") dominate, in the case of school shooters it appears that cases of murder–suicide typically involve perversions of justice and/or glory.

For example, in 2007 college student Seung–Hui Cho perpetrated 32 murders at Virginia Tech University before killing himself. Information collected on Cho after his death revealed that he was very isolated, having essentially no close friends or romantic partners. He left a suicide note in his Virginia Tech dorm room that described his classmates as "rich kids" and "deceitful charlatans" who regularly engaged in "debauchery." In his suicide note and in a video he mailed to NBC, Cho compared himself to Jesus Christ in that by killing the "rich kids" he would become "the savior of the oppressed, the downtrodden, the poor, and the rejected" (Joiner, 2014, p. 13). As Joiner (2014) notes, "in his comparison of himself to Christ, and in some of the other materials Cho sent to NBC, references to the virtue of glory can occasionally be detected. But, in Cho's mind, the reason he would receive glory is because he would deliver justice; the virtue of justice was primary for him (and grossly perverted by him)" (p. 13). Cho clearly saw his behavior as being justified, but in actuality it was clearly a perversion of justice. As a panel that investigated Cho after his rampage at Virginia Tech noted, "his thought processes were so distorted that he began arguing to himself that his *evil* plan was actually doing good" (Joiner, 2014, p. 13). If Cho's case appeared to be a perversion of glory when it was in fact primarily a perversion of justice, the opposite was the case in the Columbine tragedy. In that incident, it was widely reported in the media that Harris and Klebold were social misfits who wanted to take revenge on a number of student athletes who had bullied them. In fact, Harris in Klebold were not social misfits, they were not bullied (although they were known to bully other students), and they did not intentionally target athletes in their attack (Cullen, 2009). Instead, as their journals and videos disturbingly indicated, "their motive was a perverted version of glory and had very little to do with justice" (Joiner, 2014, p. 173). Their initial (and failed) plan was to set off a series of bombs at the school, with the goal of exceeding the death count of 168 that resulted from the Oklahoma City bombings perpetrated by Timothy McVeigh in 1995. They wanted to be remembered forever – a clear case of perverted glory (Joiner, 2014).

## GUN–RELATED VIOLENCE AND YOUTH

Gun violence is a national public health problem in the US, resulting in more than 31,000 deaths and 78,000 injuries each year (American Psychological Association, 2013). Although the rate of gun–related homicides has declined in recent years, US rates remain substantially higher than those of almost every other nation in the world (Alpers and Wilson, 2013). Moreover, although gun–related violence is often associated with homicide, suicide accounts for approximately 61% of all firearm fatalities in the US (American Psychological Association, 2013). Youth gun violence is seen as a particularly pernicious problem in the US. It is also frequently sensationalized and misunderstood, in part because of the increasingly public acts of violence and the subsequent media coverage that surrounds it, such as incidents of school shootings (American Psychological Association, 2013). In fact, only a small number of youthful offenders commit the majority of violent juvenile crimes in the US (Williams, Tuthill, and Lio, 2008). Moreover, as noted earlier, schools are among the safest places for children to be, and only a very small percentage of gun violence occurs within or near schools. That said, when life-threatening violence does occur in schools – whether it is attempted murder, murder, suicide, or murder–suicide – a gun is almost always involved. Furthermore, guns provide individuals who use them with the means to carry out multiple–fatality shootings that result not only in injuries and death but also in severe trauma and grief across schools and communities (American Psychological Association, 2013).

## A PUBLIC HEALTH APPROACH TO GUN–RELATED VIOLENCE IN SCHOOLS

The lack of ability to predict with precision which individuals will become violent has led some individuals to question whether preventing gun violence, whether in schools or elsewhere, is even possible. This is a common misconception, because effective prevention does not require prediction of specific individual behavior (American Psychological Association, 2013). Instead, the most effective prevention models target entire populations in what has become known as a public health approach. Public health models first gained notoriety in the 19$^{th}$ century, when physicians and government officials began considering the ways in which various societal and environmental variables were causing, contributing to, and/or exacerbating particular health conditions (Doll and Cummings, 2008).

Many public health initiatives have been successfully implemented since that time, especially in the last few decades. For example, public health campaigns have reduced problems ranging from lung cancer to motor vehicle accidents by accurately identifying risk factors and promoting safer behavior, even though it is not possible to predict whether a specific individual will develop lung cancer or experience a motor vehicle accident (Mozaffarian, Hemenway, and Ludwig, 2013).Public health models have also been used successfully for variety of academic, social, emotional, and behavioral problems in schools (Doll and Cummings, 2008; Shinn and Walker, 2010). Often referred to as the three–tier model (Shinn and Walker, 2010), public health approaches in schools typically include universal prevention strategies for entire populations of students, selected intervention strategies for at–risk students, and tertiary interventions for students currently exhibiting problems or in crisis (Miller, 2011).

A public health approach to the prevention of gun–related violence is becoming increasingly recommended (American Psychological Association, 2013; Mozaffarian et al., 2013), including gun–related violence in schools (Bondü et al., 2013).

## Universal Prevention Strategies

Universal prevention strategies seek to limit the influence of risk factors and strengthen protective factors in the general population before any negative developments or significant problems are observed (Bondü et al., 2013). The prevention strategies are "universal" in the sense that everyone in a particular population (e.g., entire school district, entire school, entire grade level, entire classroom) receives the intervention. Universal strategies for school shootings are frequently focused on preventing aggressive and violent behavior among children and adolescents generally. Some examples of possible universal prevention strategies in schools and communities are described below.

## Promote Gun Safety and Restrict Access to Guns

One of the most important methods for preventing youth gun violence is to promote gun safety and restrict access to guns by children and adolescents (American Psychological Association, 2013). Research has clearly demonstrated that many families with children own guns and do not keep them safety stored in the home (Johnson, Miller, Vriniotis, Azrael, and Hemenway, 2006). Moreover, although having firearms in the home is not a direct cause of youth gun violence, the rates of homicides, suicides, and unintentional firearm fatalities are higher for 5 to 14–year–olds who live in areas in which the rates of gun ownership are more prevalent (Miller, Azrael, and Hemenway, 2002). Additionally, parents and other family members play an important role in establishing and maintaining particular beliefs about violence and gun usage (American Psychological Association, 2013). In particular, poor parental monitoring and supervision, which are more general risk factors for involvement in violent behaviors (Dodge et al., 2008), may substantially increase the risk for youth gun violence (American Psychological Association, 2013).

The issue of promoting gun safety and restricting access to guns is particularly pertinent in cases of suicide, given that most youth who die by suicide in the US use guns as their lethal method (American Psychological Association, 2013). The presence of guns in a youth's home, especially unlocked loaded handguns, are associated with a significantly increased risk for suicide (American Psychological Association, 2013; Leenaars, 2009; Simon, 2007). Moreover, the risk resulting from guns is increased by their accessibility and number available, and if a gun is used to attempt suicide a fatal outcome will occur between 78% and 90% of the time (Berman, Jobes, and Silverman, 2006). Public policy initiatives that have restricted the access to guns are associated with a reduction in suicide by firearms and in suicide overall, especially among young people (Leenaars, 2009). Consequently, one of the most powerful youth suicide prevention strategies is removing guns from a young person's home environment (American Psychological Association, 2013; Berman et al., 2006; King, Foster, and Rogalski, 2013). School personnel are therefore encouraged to provide parents with information on effective means restriction. It is particularly important to convince parents of children deemed at–risk for suicide to remove their child's access to firearms (King et al., 2013).

Unfortunately, for well over a decade research on gun violence has been curtailed by legal restrictions, a lack of funding, and political pressure applied to agencies not to fund research on particular gun–related topics (American Psychological Association, 2013). Political pressure by groups such as the National Rifle Association (NRA) has had a particularly deleterious effect on gun violence research and has impeded the development of effective prevention programs related to gun violence.

## Limit Violent Media Consumption

Research has clearly established that repeated exposure to media violence (e.g., video games, TV, movies) can increase the likelihood of aggressive thoughts, emotions, and behavior. More specifically, exposure to media violence can lead to a number of negative outcomes, including (a) modeling inappropriate behaviors; (b) aggressive arousal; (c) increased risk–taking behavior; and (d) desensitization to the harmful effects of violence (Interdisciplinary Group on Preventing School and Community Violence, 2013).

One of the frequently found characteristics of school shooters identified by the US Secret Service and the Department of Education was that perpetrators often had a preoccupation with violent games and fantasies (Fein et al., 2002). Violent media consumption, especially violent video game consumption, is considered to be a risk factor for aggressive behavior generally, including school shootings (Verlinden, Hersen, and Thomas, 2000). Prohibiting or limiting access of youth to particularly violent video games, especially games involving the player "shooting" various video–created characters, has been suggested (Bondü et al., 2013). At the very least, schools can ensure that all parents receive information on the possible negative effects of violent media consumption and be encouraged to monitor their children's exposure to it.

That said, there is no evidence that violent entertainment, especially violent video games, are causally linked to mass murder, including school shootings (Fox and DeLateur, 2014). Moreover, "to the extent that youngsters spend endless hours being entertained by violence says more about the lack of parental supervision and control. It isn't that entertainment media are so powerful; it is that our other institutions – family, school, religion, and neighborhood – have grown weaker with respect to socializing children" (Fox and DeLateur, 2014, p. 133).

## Promote the Reporting of Suspicious Behavior

Various studies have conclusively demonstrated that school shooters often tell at least one other person, typically a peer, about their plans prior to carrying them out. Consequently, a promising universal strategy in schools would be to acknowledge this fact and encourage students to report to an adult any suspicious behavior they may observe or suspicious comments they may hear. For example, if students hear one of their peers verbalize threats to engage in a violent act or observe severe mood changes or other unusual behaviors in their peers, it would be beneficial to report that information to a trusted adult in the school or community (Interdisciplinary Group on Preventing School and Community Violence, 2013).

Comprehensive analyses by the US Secret Service, the FBI, and many researchers indicates that maintaining close communication and trust with students and others in the community is the most effective method for preventing many acts of violence targeted at schools (Interdisciplinary Group on Preventing School and Community Violence, 2013). Adults should be careful to communicate that reporting such suspicions is not "snitching" or "tattling" but rather that "their lives or the lives of their friends might depend on seeking help for troubled individuals before problems escalate" (Interdisciplinary Group on Preventing School and Community Violence, 2013, p. 121).

Moreover, because research suggests that the most common reason students do *not* report a serious threat is a fear of retaliation, school personnel may need to address these concerns when threats are brought to their attention (Nekvasil and Cornell, 2012). The probability of students reporting suspicious behavior in their peers and engaging in help–seeking can be enhanced when students have positive and mutually respectful relationships with school personnel. In fact, there have been a number of instances where students conceivably prevented school shootings when they observed suspicious behavior or learned of a possible attack and promptly reported it to appropriate adults (Daniels and Page, 2013).

**Promote Safe and Supportive Schools and a Positive School Climate**

Decades of research have yielded the consistent finding that school climate and school violence are integrally related (Gottfredson, 2001; Mayer, 2002; Osher, Dwyer, Jimerson, and Brown, 2012). Punitive school environments appear to promote antisocial behavior. Specifically, overreliance on punishment, unclear expectations of students, frequent academic failure experiences, lack of student involvement with and connectedness to the school, inconsistent consequences, and lack of administrative support of staff have been identified as key contextual factors that promote aggression and violence in the school (Mayer, 2002; Sprague and Walker, 2010). This research is so well-established that in the year 2000 the US Department of Education asserted, "Studies indicate that approximately four of every five disruptive students can be traced to some dysfunction in the ways school are organized, staff members are trained, or schools are run." (US Dept. of Education, 2000, p.10). Consequently, creating positive school climates addressing these contextual factors has been cited as a critical practice to diminish the risk of violence in schools (Eisenbraun, 2007; Mayer, 2002; Osher et al., 2012), and the US Secret Service suggests that effective threat assessment can *only* occur in a larger context of school climate and safety (Fein et al., 2002).

Comprehensive, school–wide approaches to violence prevention target all students, all staff, and all areas of the building. Although there are several empirically–supported approaches to creating positive school climates (e.g., school–wide positive behavior support, Olweus Bullying Prevention), they typically and minimally involve creating and systematically teaching clear rules to students, increasing the number of positive interactions between students and school staff (through praise and often more structured positive consequence systems), decreasing reliance on reactive punitive strategies to remediate more mild behavior problems, and matching student skill with instructional level (Limber, 2012; Mayer, 2002; Sprague and Horner, 2012). Research demonstrates that when schools implement these practices with integrity, particularly over time, they achieve outcomes such as fewer referrals to the office, fewer instances of assault and vandalism, decreased suspensions and expulsions, improved staff and student perceptions of being safe (Limber, 2011; Mayer, 2002; Sprague and Horner 2012), and increased academic achievement (Brennan, 2013).

To better promote school safety, each student should have a positive, ongoing connection to at least one adult in a position of authority (Fein et al.,

2002; Maynard, Kjellstrand, and Thompson, 2014). This is recommended to help offset the risk of students engaging in antisocial behavior and also increase the likelihood that students will share their concerns and any warning signs they observe in their peers (i.e., break the culture of silence). In order to reach all students, Fein et al. (2002) suggest that schools take concrete steps to identify and work with students who have few connections to the school. For example, during a faculty meeting staff could be asked to put stars next to the names of students with whom they have the closest relationships. School personnel would then make active attempts to increase positive contact with students who were not initially identified.

## Selected and Indicated Strategies

Selected strategies refer to interventions for individuals who may be at–risk for a particular problem, whereas indicated strategies are utilized when an individual is at high-risk for problems or already exhibiting them (Miller, 2011). For some problems, the application of selected and indicated strategies function on a continuum and may overlap, given that "at-risk" individuals can quickly become "high-risk" individuals in certain situations. This can occur, for example, when a particular student engages in threatening behavior of some kind, such as "leaking" his intentions to peers about bringing a gun to school. In such situations, a thorough threat assessment should be conducted on the student, and it may be useful to supplement it with a suicide risk assessment as well. Both of these assessment strategies are discussed below.

### Threat Assessment

As previously discussed in this chapter, there is no typical profile of a school shooter. School shooters have varied widely in terms of age, racial and ethnic background, social centrality, socioeconomic status, academic achievement, and family situation. However, there is a clear and consistent process, or pattern of behavior, undertaken by most school shooters. Specifically, most attackers (a) formed a plan at least two weeks in advance, (b) communicated their plan with at least one other person (typically a peer), (c) went through a process of acquiring firearms, most often from their home, and (d) displayed behavior that signaled problems coping and feelings of helplessness (e.g., suicidal behavior, writing about suicide and/or homicide) which led others to be concerned (Borum et al., 2010; Fein, 2002; National Institute of Justice, 2002). In addition, revenge against specific students and/or administrators was a motive in the majority of school shootings, and in many cases the attacker had a long history of being bullied and harassed (National Institute of Justice, 2002).

The purpose of threat assessment is to identify students who pose a risk of engaging in a school shooting, determine the level of threat, and intervene as early as possible in the intent–planning–preparation process outlined above. The FBI report *The School Shooter: A Threat Assessment Perspective* (O'Toole, 2000) and US Secret Service report *Threat Assessment in Schools: A Guide to Managing Threatening Situations and to Creating Safe School Climates* (Fein et al., 2002), both available to the public online, provide comprehensive models for assessment. Broadly, according to these sources threat assessment is conceptualized on a continuum in which there are two phases: threat assessment *inquiry* and threat assessment *investigation*. Threat assessment *inquiry* is typically conducted by school personnel and is geared towards gathering information that can be obtained at school or by people associated with the school. Part of the inquiry is evaluating direct threats and leakage. (For example, the school team examines the types of any verbal threats made, the emotional content of threats, specific, plausible details of a plan, and whether steps have been taken to carry out a plan.) If the inquiry suggests a student is seriously considering an attack and/or any violation of law has occurred, then the process of a threat assessment *investigation*, conducted by law enforcement agencies, would be undertaken.

The goals of both threat assessment inquiry and investigation are to determine the level of targeted risk; an additional goal of threat assessment investigation is to determine if any laws have been or likely will be broken. Both types of assessment also take into consideration four key variables or assessment "prongs": (1) the behavior of the student (e.g., leakage, poor coping skills, signs of depression, spending unusual amounts of time practicing with firearms), (2) family dynamics (e.g., access to weapons, parental acceptance of child pathological behavior, few or no limits on child by parents), (3) school dynamics and the student's role in those dynamics (e.g., student lack of connectedness to school, school tolerance of bullying, inequitable discipline), and (4) social dynamics (e.g., peer groups who share a fascination with violence, drugs and alcohol, copycat effect of school shootings and suicides). Following a threat assessment inquiry and/or investigation, the student's level of assessed threat, or risk to the safety of others, dictates intervention at the school and/or law enforcement level. Also occurring along a continuum, threat management (i.e., intervention) includes but is not limited to taking no action, referring a student for counseling, school disciplinary response, student hospitalization, notification to the student body of a threat, emergency response procedures, and/or student arrest (Fein et al., 2002; O'Toole, 2000).

The FBI and Secret Service reports note that to use the threat assessment model effectively those conducting the assessment should have appropriate training (Fein et al., 2002; O'Toole, 2000). However, at the time of these reports, schools had little to no training with this approach and ways in which to practically implement the model were not clear (Cornell, 2013). In response, researchers at the University of Virginia developed a set of guidelines designed to help school personnel, mental health staff, and law enforcement assess and respond to threats in Kindergarten through 12$^{th}$ grade. Specifically, threat assessment teams are trained in the Virginia Student Threat Assessment Guidelines (V-STAG) via a six–hour workshop that prepares them to use the 145–page threat assessment manual (Cornell, 2013; Cornell and Sheras, 2006).

Broadly, V-STAG is a three– to six–step assessment and intervention process, depending on whether the threat is deemed transient (i.e., remarks reflect temporary feelings of anger or frustration without any intent to harm; often resolved immediately with an apology) or substantive (i.e., remarks reflect intent to physically injure someone beyond the immediate situation; protective action is necessary and law enforcement action may be required). In moving through the assessment process, the threat assessment team considers facts such as student age, capability to carry out the threat, discipline history, credibility of the threat, credibility of witness accounts, and willingness to acknowledge behavior (Cornell and Sheras, 2006). The cost of V–STAG to the district is currently $4000 for team training, which includes three hours of follow–up consultation and $45 for the cost of the book (SAMHSA Intervention Summary – Virginia Student Threat Assessment Guidelines, n.d.). Use of the V-STAG has been associated with long-term reductions in school suspensions and expulsions (Cornell, Allen, and Fan, 2012; Cornell, Gregory, and Fan, 2011), decreased bullying infractions in school (Cornell, Sheras, Gregory, and Fan, 2009), and improved school climate (Cornell et al., 2009). In addition, school personnel trained in V-STAG reported a substantial decrease in concerns about school homicide following training in the threat assessment approach (Korrie, Cornell, Lorek, and Sheras, 2008).

## Suicide Risk Assessment

Given that many individuals who pose a threat to others also frequently pose a threat to themselves, students for whom a threat assessment is conducted should generally also be assessed for their potential risk for suicide. The issues that should be considered in conducting a thorough suicide risk assessment are complex and nuanced, and space limitations preclude a thorough discussion of these issues in this chapter. However, as a general rule, individuals conducting suicide risk assessments should be cognizant of four basic principles (King et al., 2013). First, these individuals should be aware that the risk for suicide can be adequately understood and conceptualized. Substantial research conducted over many years has repeatedly demonstrated that there are clear and consistent risk factors for suicide, including previous suicide attempts, clinical depression, and alcohol abuse. Second, the risk for suicide is not static, and therefore assessment of suicide risk must be ongoing. Third, the risk for suicide is not always conspicuous. That is, individuals who are suicidal may not choose to share information about their suicidal thoughts, impulses, or plans with parents, school personnel, or mental health professionals. Finally, a comprehensive suicide risk assessment is best facilitated through the use of multiple informants (King et al., 2013).

All students who are considered potentially at risk for suicidal behavior should be individually interviewed by a school–based mental health professional (e.g., school psychologist) who is adequately trained in suicide risk assessment. Examples of areas that should be explored with at-risk students include (a) how the student currently feels; (b) past and current levels of depression, hopelessness, and suicidal ideation; (c) perceptions of possible burdensomeness and disconnection to others; (d) a history of any previous suicidal behavior, particularly suicide attempts; (e) the presence or absence of a suicide plan; (f) the degree of specificity and lethality of method in the suicide plan; (g) availability of lethal methods; (h) possibility of rescue; (i) current support systems; and (j) reasons to live (Miller, 2011, 2013). In addition, mental health professionals should assess possible imminent warning signs for suicide (some of which can be directly observed), including agitation, insomnia, nightmares, and social withdrawal (Joiner, 2014).

Given that a high percentage of school shooters were known to have been suicidal, an adequate understanding of suicide and how to prevent it is critical. In his examination of murder–suicide, Joiner (2014) provided compelling evidence that suicide is the primary motivation of perpetrators, and that effective suicide prevention is also effective murder–suicide prevention.

Consequently, effective suicide prevention should be viewed as an integral component of preventing school shootings. A comprehensive discussion of effective school–based suicide prevention programs, including universal strategies, selected and indicated strategies, and postvention procedures, is outside the scope of this chapter. Readers interested in additional information on these topics are referred to Eklund and Gueldner (2012), Hart (2012), King et al., (2013), Miller (2011, 2012 a,b, 2013), and Miller and Mazza (2013, in press).

## Crisis Intervention Strategies

Crisis prevention and intervention has become an increasingly important activity in schools (Brock and Jimerson, 2012; Brock et al., 2009; Nickerson et al., 2014), including the prevention of school violence (Brock, Jimerson, Hart, and Nickerson, 2009; Jimerson, Nickerson, Mayer, and Furlong, 2012) and responding effectively to sudden and unexpected deaths in schools (Jimerson, Brown, and Stewart, 2012). Unfortunately, empirical evidence to guide school personnel in developing and implementing effective crisis response procedures for school shootings is lacking (Borum et al., 2010). School personnel must currently rely upon on the insights generated from emergency management strategies used in community workplace settings as well as lessons learned in the aftermath of school shootings (Borum et al., 2010; Crepeau–Hobson, Sievering, Armstrong, and Stonis, 2012). There is considerable variation, however, between schools in terms of the support services they provide for students, school personnel, and families in the aftermath of a school shooting (Borum et al., 2010). Developing and maintaining effective crisis services in schools is critical, as is having a cadre of trained, experienced professionals who can quickly converge to provide effective crisis intervention (Borum et al., 2010).

One example of a school–based crisis prevention and intervention program that may be useful in the context of school shootings is PREPaRE (Brock et al., 2009; Brock, Jimerson, Hart, and Nickerson, 2012). Developed through the collaborative efforts of workgroups sponsored by the National Association of School Psychologists (NASP) specifically for school–based mental health professionals, PREPaRE incorporates recommendations for crisis teams offered by the US Department of Education and the US Department of Homeland Security, as well as research and scholarship on effective emergency preparedness and crisis response (Brock et al., 2009).

The PREPaRE model acronym specifies a hierarchical and sequential set of activities, including *P*reventing and preparing for psychological trauma; *R*eaffirming physical health and perceptions of security and safety; *E*valuating psychological trauma risk; *P*roviding interventions *a*nd *R*esponding to psychological needs; and *E*xamining the effectiveness of crisis prevention and intervention (Brock et al., 2009). Although research examining the effectiveness of the PREPaRE model is in its early stages, there are indications that school–based mental health professionals trained in PREPaRE report significant improvements in crisis prevention and intervention attitudes and knowledge (Brock et al., 2012; Nickerson et al., 2014).

In effectively responding to a school shooting, there is first and foremost an immediate need to communicate and collaborate with local emergency responders (Borum et al., 2010). The PREPaRE model emphasizes planning with local law enforcement and emergency medical personnel to establish a clear understanding of the roles of each during a crisis. In addition, PREPaRE describes specific responses to support students and school personnel immediately following a crisis event such as a school shooting, including reaffirming physical health and perceptions of safety, evaluating factors that increase the risk of developing psychological trauma, and providing crisis interventions to address individual needs (Borum et al., 2010; Brock et al., 2009, 2012).

Borum and his colleagues (2010) also suggest that it might be beneficial to examine current best practices in disaster mental health to determine if these might be relevant to a post–shooting response, given that more research and infrastructure development has been devoted to mental health responses to natural disasters than to school shootings.

Although community–based emergency responders will be needed in cases involving school shootings, school personnel have an equally important role in this process. Emergency preparedness and pre–crisis planning are essential, as "an effective response is contingent on school personnel receiving training in crisis response" (Crepeau–Hobson et al., 2012. p. 209). School crisis response teams – typically composed of a school psychologist, school counselor, school nurse, school administrator, teachers, and support staff – will require adequate training in threat assessment as well as other aspects of crisis prevention and intervention (Crepeau–Hobson et al., 2012). Although turf issues may develop and need to be addressed, creating a district–level crisis response team may be beneficial as well, especially given that site–based crisis response teams frequently are overwhelmed in cases of school shootings (Adamson and Peacock, 2007).

Having a designated mental health incident commander (MHIC) or point person to lead the team(s) and quickly make response–related decisions is another critical component of an effective crisis response (Crepeau–Hobson et al., 2012).

Finally, school personnel should work closely with emergency responders in terms of emergency preparedness to ensure adequate communication and coordination of services. For example, many school districts do not appear to have detailed blueprints of their school building and facilities readily available to local police (Dumitriu, 2013).

This is critically important, given that when a school shooting occurs the first priority for law enforcement is an action plan to enter the school, evacuate students and school personnel, and stop the attack as quickly as possible. For example, one of the SWAT teams that entered Columbine High School after the school shootings that occurred there had to request a floor plan of the school when they were unable to find the school library, which contained several injured students (Dumitriu, 2013). The longer the interval between school shootings and the evacuation of victims, the more likely serious injuries and death will result.

## CONCLUSION

School shootings are very rare but extremely horrific and tragic events. A public health approach in both schools and communities may be useful in preventing school shootings, but this will require the coordinated efforts of schools, colleges and universities, law enforcement, and other emergency responders. Interventions that may prove particularly useful in efforts to prevent school shootings include promoting gun safety and restricting access to guns among young people, particularly those at–risk; creating school and community cultures in which young people feel comfortable approaching adults when they suspect one of their peers may be potentially dangerous; training school–based mental health professionals in threat assessment; engaging in effective emergency preparedness in both schools and communities; and responding quickly and effectively when a crisis occurs to minimize injuries and loss of life.

## REFERENCES

Adamson, A. D. and Peacock, G. G. (2007). Crisis response in the public schools: A survey of school psychologists' experiences and perceptions. *Psychology in the Schools,* 44, 749-764.

Alpers, P. and Wilson, M. (2013). *Global impact of gun violence: Firearms, public health and safety.* Retrieved from http://www.gunpolicy.org/firearms/region.

American Psychological Association. (1999). *Warning signs: A violence prevention guide for youth.* Retrieved from http://helping.apa.org/warningsigns/index.html.

American Psychological Association. (2013). *Gun violence: Prediction, prevention, and policy.* Available at http://www.apa.org/pubs/info/reports/gun-violence-prevention.aspx.

American Psychological Association Zero Tolerance Task Force. (2008). Are zero tolerance policies effective in the schools? An evidentiary review and recommendations. *American Psychologist,* 63, 852-862.

Bachman, R., Randolph, A. and Brown, B. L. (2011). Predicting perceptions of fear at school and going to and from school for African American and White students: The effects of school security measures. *Youth and Society,* 43, 705-726.

Band, S. R. and Harpold, J. A. (1999, September). School violence: Lessons learned. *FBI: Law Enforcement Bulletin,* 68, 9-16.

Berman, A. L., Jobes, D. A. and Silverman, M. M. (2006). *Adolescent suicide: Assessment and intervention, second edition.* Washington, DC: American Psychological Association.

Böckler, N., Seeter, T., Sitzer, P., and Heitmeyer, W. (2013a). (Eds.). *School shootings: International research, case studies, and concepts for prevention.* New York, NY: Springer.

Böckler, N., Seeger, T., Sitzer, P., and Heitmeyer, W. (2013b). School shootings: Conceptual framework and international empirical trends. In: N. Böckler, T. Seeger, P. Sitzer, and W. Heitmeyer (Eds.), *School shootings: International research, case studies, and concepts for prevention* (pp. 1-24). New York, NY: Springer.

Bondü, R., Scheithauer, H., Leuschner, V., and Cornell, D. G. (2013). International perspectives on prevention and intervention in school shootings. In: N. Böckler, T. Seeger, P. Sitzer, and W. Heitmeyer (Eds.), *School shootings: International research, case studies, and concepts for prevention* (pp. 343-362). New York, NY: Springer.

Borum, R., Cornell, D. G., Modzeleski, W., and Jimerson, S. R. (2010). What can be done about school shootings?: A review of the evidence. *Educational Researcher,* 39, 27-37.

Brennan, L. M., Shelleby, E. C., Shaw, D. S., Gardner, F., Dishion, T. J., and Wilson, M. (2013). Indirect effects of the family check-up on school-age academic achievement through improvements in parenting in early childhood. *Journal of Educational Psychology,* 105, 762-773.

Brock, S. E. and Jimerson, S. R. (Eds.). (2012). *Best practices in school crisis prevention and intervention, second edition.* Bethesda, MD: National Association of School Psychologists.

Brock, S. E., Jimerson, S. R., Hart, S. R., and Nickerson, A. B. (2012). Preventing, preparing for, and responding to school violence with the PREPaRE model. In: S. R. Jimerson, A. B. Nickerson, M. J. Mayer, and M. J. Furlong (Eds.), *Handbook of school violence and school safety: International research and practice, second edition* (pp. 463-474). New York, NY: Routledge.

Brock, S. E., Nickerson, A. B., Reeves, M. A., Jimerson, S. R., Lieberman, R. A., and Feinberg, T. A. (2009). *School crisis prevention and intervention: The PREPaRE model.* Bethesda, MD: National Association of School Psychologists.

Cornell, D. (2006). *School violence: Fears versus facts.* Mahwah, NJ: Lawrence Erlbaum.

Cornell, D. (2013). The Virginia student threat assessment guidelines: An empirically supported violence prevention strategy. In: N. Böckler, T. Seeger, P. Sitzer, and W. Heitmeyer (Eds.), *School shootings: International research, case studies, and concepts for prevention* (pp. 379-400).

Cornell, D. G., Allen, K. and Fan, X. (2012). A randomized controlled study of the Virginia Student Threat Assessment Guidelines in kindergarten through grade 12. *School Psychology Review,* 41, 100-115.

Cornell, D. G., Gregory, A. and Fan, X. (2011). Reductions in long–term suspensions following adoption of adoption of the Virginia student threat assessment guidelines. *NASSP Bulletin,* 95, 175-194.

Cornell, D. and Nekvasil, E. (2012). Violent thoughts and behaviors. In: S. E. Brock and S. R. Jimerson (Eds.), *Best practices in school crisis prevention and intervention* (pp. 485-502). Bethesda, MD: National Association of School Psychologists.

Cornell, D. and Sheras, P. (2006). *Guidelines for responding to student threats of violence*. Longmont, CO: Sopris West.

Cornell, D., Sheras, P., Gregory, A., and Fan, X. (2009). A retrospective study of school safety conditions in high schools using the Virginia Threat Assessment Guidelines versus alternative approaches. *School Psychology Quarterly,* 24, 119-129.

Crepeau–Hobson, F., Sievering, K. S., Armstrong, C., and Stonis, J. (2012). A coordinated mental health crisis response: Lessons learned from three Colorado school shootings. *Journal of School Violence,* 11, 207-225.

Cullen, D. (2009). *Columbine.* New York, NY: Twelve.

Daniels, J. A. and Page, J. W. (2013). Averted school shootings. In: N. Böckler, T. Seeger, P. Sitzer, and W. Heitmeyer (Eds.), *School shootings: International research, case studies, and concepts for prevention* (pp. 421-439). New York, NY: Springer.

Dinkes, R., Cataldi, E. F. and Lin–Kelly, W. (2007). *Indicators of school crime and safety: 2007 (NCES 2008–021/NCJ 219553).* Washington, DC: National Center for Education Statistics, Institute of Education Sciences, US Department of Education and Bureau of Justice Statistics, Office of Justice Programs, US Department of Justice.

Dodge, K. A., Greenberg, M. T., Malone, P. S., and Conduct Problems Prevention Research Group. (2008). Testing an idealized dynamic cascade model of the development of serious violence in adolescents. *Child Development,* 79, 1907-1927.

Doll, B. and Cummings, J. A. (Eds.). (2008). *Transforming school mental health services: Population–based approaches to promoting the competency and wellness of children.* Thousand Oaks, CA: Corwin Press.

Dumitriu, C. (2013). Crisis management in school shooting situations: The school – A forgotten fact in the equation. In: N. Böckler, T. Seeger, P. Sitzer, and W. Heitmeyer (Eds.), *School shootings: International research, case studies, and concepts for prevention* (pp. 441-476). New York, NY: Springer.

Dwyer, K., Osher, D. and Warger, C. (1998). *Early warning, timely response: A guide to safe schools.* Washington, DC: US Department of Education.

Eisenbraun, K. D. (2007). Violence in schools: Prevalence, prediction, and prevention. *Aggression and Violent Behavior,* 12, 459-469.

Eklund, K. and Gueldner, B. (2012). Suicidal thoughts and behaviors: Suicide intervention. In: S. E. Brock and S. R. Jimerson (Eds.), *Best practices in school crisis prevention and intervention, second edition* (pp. 503-523). Bethesda, MD: National Association of School Psychologists.

Fein, R., Vossekuil, B., Pollack, W., Borum, R., Modzeleski, W., and Reddy, M. (2002). *Threat assessment in schools: A guide to managing threatening situations and to creating safe school climates.* Washington, DC: US Secret Service and Department of Education.

Fox, J. A. and DeLateur, M. J. (2014). Mass shootings in America: Moving beyond Newtown. *Homicide Studies,* 18, 125-145.

Furlong, M., Bates, M. and Smith, D. (2001). Predicting school weapon possession: A secondary analysis of the Youth Risk Behavior Surveillance Survey. *Psychology in the Schools,* 38, 127-140.

Furlong, M. J., Sharkey, J. D., Bates, M. P., and Smith, D. C. (2004). An examination of the reliability, data screening procedures, and extreme response patterns for the Youth Risk Behavior Surveillance Survey. *Journal of School Violence,* 3, 109-130.

Gill, M. and Sprigs, A. (2005). *Assessing the impact of CCTV.* London: Home Office Research, Development and Statistics Directorate.

Gottfredson, D. C. (2001). *Schools and delinquency.* New York, NY: Cambridge University Press.

Grant, E. (2003). Making schools safe for the 21st century: An interview with Ronald D. Stephens. *Educational Forum,* 67, 156-162.

Grossman, D. (1995). *On killing: The psychological cost of learning to kill in war and society.* Boston, MA: Back Bay Books.

Hart, S. R. (2012). Student suicide: Suicide postvention. In: S. E. Brock and S. R. Jimerson (Eds.), *Best practices in school crisis prevention and intervention, second edition* (pp. 525-547). Bethesda, MD: National Association of School Psychologists.

Heilbrun, K., Dvoskin, J. and Heilbrun, A. (2009). Toward preventing future tragedies: Mass killings on college campuses, public health, and threat/ risk assessment. *Psychological Inquiring and Law,* 2, 93-99.

Interdisciplinary Group on Preventing School and Community Violence (2013). December 2012 Connecticut school shooting position statement. *Journal of School Violence,* 12, 119-133.

Jimerson, S. R., Brown, J. A. and Stewart, K. T. (2012). Sudden and unexpected student death: Preparing for and responding to the unpredictable. In: S. E. Brock and S. R. Jimerson (Eds.), *Best practices in school crisis prevention and intervention, second edition* (pp. 469-483). Bethesda, MD: National Association of School Psychologists.

Jimerson, S. R., Hart, S. R. and Renshaw, T. L. (2012). Conceptual foundations for understanding youth engaged in antisocial and aggressive behaviors. In: S. R. Jimerson, A. B. Nickerson, M. J. Mayer, and M. J. Furlong (Eds.), *Handbook of school violence and school safety:*

*International research and practice, second edition* (pp. 3-14). New York, NY: Routledge.

Jimerson, S. R., Nickerson, A. B., Mayer, M. J., and Furlong, M. J. (Eds.). (2012). *Handbook of school violence and school safety: International research and practice, second edition.* New York, NY: Routledge.

Johnson, R. M., Miller, M., Vriniotis, M., Azrael, D., and Hemenway, D. (2006). Are household firearms stored less safely in homes with adolescents? Analysis of a national random sample of parents. *Archives of Pediatric and Adolescent Medicine,* 160, 788-792.

Joiner, T. (2005). *Why people die by suicide.* Cambridge, MA: Harvard University Press.

Joiner, T. (2014). *The perversion of virtue: Understanding murder–suicide.* New York, NY: Oxford University Press.

King, C. A., Foster, C. E. and Rogalski, K. M. (2013). *Teen suicide risk: A practitioner guide to screening, assessment, and management.* New York, NY: Guilford.

Korrie, A., Cornell, D., Lorek, E., and Sheras, P. (2008). Response of school personnel to student threat assessment training. *School Effectiveness and School Improvement,* 19, 319-332.

Langman, P. (2009a). Rampage school shooters: A typology. *Aggression and Violent Behavior,* 14, 79-86.

Langman, P. (2009b). *Why kids kill: Inside the minds of school shooters.* New York, NY: Palgrave Macmillan.

Langman, P. (2013). Thirty–five rampage school shooters: Trends, patterns, and typology. In: N. Böckler, T. Seeger, P. Sitzer, and W. Heitmeyer (Eds.), *School shootings: International research, case studies, and concepts for prevention* (pp. 131-156). New York, NY: Springer.

Lankford, A. (2013). *The myth of martyrdom: What really drives suicide bombers, rampage shooters, and other self–destructive killers.* New York, NY: Palgrave Macmillan.

Lankford, A., and Hakim, N. (2011). From Columbine to Palestine: A comparative analysis of rampage shooters in the United States and volunteer suicide bombers in the Middle East. *Aggression and Violent Behavior,* 16, 98-107.

Leenaars, A. (2009). Gun availability and control in suicide prevention. In: D. Wasserman and C. Wasserman (Eds.), *Oxford textbook of suicidology and suicide prevention* (pp. 577-581). New York, NY: Oxford University Press.

Limber, S. P. (2011). Development, evaluation, and future directions of the Olweus Bullying Prevention Program. *Journal of School Violence,* 10, 71-87.

Limber, S. P. (2012). The Olweus Bullying Prevention Program: An overview of its implementation and research basis. In: S. R. Jimerson, A. B. Nickerson, M. J. Mayer, and M. J. Furlong (Eds.), *Handbook of school violence and school safety: International research and practice*, second edition (pp. 369-382). New York, NY: Routledge.

Lubell, K. M. and Vetter, J. B. (2006). Suicide and youth violence prevention: The promise of an integrated approach. *Aggression and Violent Behavior,* 11, 167-175.

Mayer, G. R. (2002). Behavioral strategies to reduce school violence. *Child and Family Behavior Therapy,* 24, 83-100.

Mayer, M. J. (2010). Structural Analysis of 1995-2005 School Crime Supplement datasets: Factors influencing students' fear, anxiety, and avoidant behaviors. *Journal of School Violence,* 9, 37-55.

Mayer, M. J. and Leone, P. E. (1999). A structural analysis of school violence and disruption: Implications for creating safer schools. *Education and Treatment of Children,* 22, 333-358.

Mayer, M. J. and Leone, P. E. (2007). School violence and disruption revisited: Equity and safety in the school house. *Focus on Exceptional Children,* 40, 1-28.

Maynard, B. R., Kjellstrand, E. K. and Thompson, A. M. (2014). Effects of check and connect on attendance, behavior, and academics: A randomized effectiveness trial. *Research on Social Work Practice,* 24, 296-309.

McGee, K. and DeBernardo, C. (1999). The classroom avenger: A behavioral profile of school based schootings. *Forensic Examiner,* 8, 16-18.

Meloy, J. R., Hoffmann, J., Roshdi, K., and Guldimann, A. (2014). Some warning behaviors discriminate between school shooters and other students of concern. *Journal of Threat Assessment and Management,* 1, 203-211.

Miller, D. N. (2011). *Child and adolescent suicidal behavior: School–based prevention, assessment, and intervention.* New York, NY: Guilford.

Miller, D. N. (2012a). Youth suicidal behavior in the context of school violence. In: S. R. Jimerson, A. B. Nickerson, M. J. Mayer, and M. J. Furlong (Eds.), *Handbook of school violence and school safety: International research and practice, second edition* (pp. 203-214). New York, NY: Routledge.

Miller, D. N. (2012b). Preventing student suicide. In: S. E. Brock and S. R. Jimerson (Eds.), *Best practices school crisis prevention and intervention, second edition* (pp. 203-222). Bethesda, MD: National Association of School Psychologists.

Miller, D. N. (2013). Assessing risk for suicide. In: S. H. McConaughy, *Clinical interviews for children and adolescents: Assessment to intervention, second edition* (pp. 208-227). New York, NY: Guilford.

Miller, D. N. and Mazza, J. J. (2013). Suicide prevention programs in schools. In: D. Lester and J. R. Rogers (Eds.), *Suicide: A global issue, volume 2: Prevention* (pp. 109-134). Santa Barbara, CA: Praeger.

Miller, D. N. and Mazza, J. J. (in press). Interventions for suicidal behavior. In: L. A. Theodore (Ed.), *The handbook of applied interventions for children and adolescents.* New York, NY: Springer.

Miller, M., Azrael, D. and Hemenway, D. (2002). Firearm availability and unintentional firearm death, suicide, and homicide among 5–14 year olds. *Journal of Trauma,* 52, 267-275.

Mozaffarian, D., Hemenway, D. and Ludwig, D. S. (2013). Curbing gun violence: Lessons from public health success. *JAMA: Journal of the American Medical Association,* 309, 551-552.

Mulvey, E. P. and Cauffman, E. (2001). The inherent limits of predicting school violence. *American Psychologist,* 56, 797-802.

National Institute of Justice. (2002). Preventing school shootings: A summary of a US Secret Service safe school initiative report. *NIJ Journal,* 248, 10-15.

Nekvasil, E. K. and Cornell, D. G. (2012). Student reports of peer threats of violence: Prevalence and outcomes. *Journal of School Violence,* 11, 357-375.

Nickerson, A. B., Serwacki, M. L., Brock, S. E., Savage, T. A., Woitaszewski, S. A., and Reeves, M. A. (2014). Program evaluation of the PREPaRE School Crisis Prevention and Intervention Training Curriculum. *Psychology in the Schools,* 51, 466-479.

Nickerson, A. B. and Slater, E. D. (2009). School and community violence and victimization as predictors of adolescent suicidal behavior. *School Psychology Review,* 38, 218-232.

Osher, D., Dwyer, K. P., Jimerson, S. R., and Brown, J. A. (2012). Developing safe, supportive, and effective schools: Facilitating student success to reduce school violence. In: S. R. Jimerson, A. B. Nickerson, M. J. Mayer, and M. J. Furlong (Eds.), *Handbook of school violence and school safety:*

*International research and practice*, second edition (pp. 27-44). New York, NY: Routledge.

O'Toole, M. E. (2000). *The school shooter: A threat assessment perspective.* Quantico, VA: National Center for the Analysis of Violent Crime, Federal Bureau of Investigation.

Owen, D. (2004). *Criminal minds: The science and psychology of profiling.* New York, NY: Barnes and Noble.

Perumean-Chaney, S. E. and Sutton, L. M. (2013). Students and perceived school safety: The impact of school security measures. *American Journal of Criminal Justice,* 38, 570-588.

Preti, A. (2008). School shooting as a culturally enforced way of expressing suicidal hostile intentions. *The Journal of the American Academy of Psychiatry and the Law,* 36, 544-550.

Priks, M. (2008, April). *Do surveillance cameras affect unruly behavior? A close look at grandstands (CESifo Working Paper Series No. 2289).* Available at SSRN:http//ssrn.com/abstract=1126633.

Raffaele–Mendez, L. M. (2003). Predictors of suspension and negative school outcomes: A longitudinal investigation. In: J. Wald and D. J. Losen (Eds.), *New directions for youth development* (no. 99; Deconstructing the school–to–prison pipeline; pp. 17-34). San Francisco, CA: Jossey–Bass.

SAMHSA Intervention Summary – Virginia Student Threat Assessment Guidelines. (n.d.). Retrieved December 15, 2014, from http://www.nrepp.samhsa.gov/ViewIntervention.aspx?id=263.

Sewell, K. W. and Mendelsohn, M. (2000). Profiling potentially violent youth: Statistical and conceptual problems. *Children's Services: Social Policy, Research, and Practice,* 3, 147-169.

Shinn, M. R. and Walker, H. M. (Eds.). (2010). *Interventions for achievement and behavior problems in a three–tier model including RTI.* Bethesda, MD: National Association of School Psychologists.

Simon, R. I. (2007). Gun safety management for patients at risk for suicide. *Suicide and Life–Threatening Behavior,* 37, 518-526.

Skiba, R. J., Shure, L. A., Middelberg, L. V., and Baker, T. L. (2012). Reforming school discipline and reducing disproportionality in suspension and expulsion. In: S. R. Jimerson, A. B. Nickerson, M. J. Mayer, and M. J. Furlong (Eds.), *Handbook of school violence and school safety: International research and practice, second edition* (pp. 515-528). New York, NY: Routledge.

Sprague, J. R. and Horner, R. H. (2012). School-wide positive behavioral intervention and supports: Proven practices and future directions. In: S. R.

Jimerson, A. B. Nickerson, M. J. Mayer, and M. J. Furlong (Eds.), *Handbook of school violence and school safety: International research and practice*, second edition (pp. 436-446). New York, NY: Routledge.

Sprague, J. R. and Walker, H. M. (2010). Building safe and healthy schools to promote school success: Critical issues, current challenges, and promising approaches. In: M. R. Shinn and H. M. Walker (Eds.), *Interventions for achievement and behavior problems in a three-tier model including RTI* (pp. 225-258). Bethesda, MD: National Association of School Psychologists.

Theriot, M. T. (2009). School resource officers and the criminalization of student behavior. *Journal of Criminal Justice,* 37, 280-287.

US Department of Education (2000). *Preventing bullying: A manual for schools and communities.* Washington, D.C.

Van Rompay, T., Vonk, D. and Fransen, M. (2009). The eye of the camera: Effects of security cameras on prosocial behavior. *Environment and Behavior,* 41, 60-74.

Verlinden, S., Hersen, M. and Thomas, J. (2000). Risk factors in school shootings. *Clinical Psychology Review,* 20, 3-56.

Vossekuil, B., Fein, R. A., Reddy, M., Borum, R., and Modzeleski, W. (2002). *The final report and findings of the Safe School Initiative: Implications for the prevention of school attacks in the United States.* Washington, DC: Secret Service and US Department of Education.

Welsh, B. and Farrington, D. (2002). *Crime prevention effects of closed circuit television: A systematic review.* London: Home Office Research, Development and Statistics Directorate.

Welsh, B. and Farrington, D. (2004). Evidence–based crime prevention: The effectiveness of CCTV. *Crime Prevention and Community Safety: An International Journal,* 6, 21-33.

Williams, K. R., Tuthill, L. and Lio, S. (2008). A portrait of juvenile offending in the United States. In: R. D. Hoge, N. G. Guerra and P. Boxer (Eds.), *Treating the juvenile offender* (pp. 15-32). New York, NY: Guilford.

In: Public Health and Harm Reduction
Editor: Meredith B. Morris
ISBN: 978-1-63482-159-9


*Chapter 2*

# ENLARGING THE SOCIAL DEFINITION OF HARM TO INCLUDE GENETICS

***Stephen M. Modell[1,2], Sharon L. R. Kardia[2] and Toby Citrin[1]***

[1]Department of Health Management and Policy, University of Michigan School of Public Health, Ann Arbor, MI, US
[2]Department of Epidemiology, University of Michigan School of Public Health, Ann Arbor, MI, US

## ABSTRACT

Harm can be both physical and social, a function of the health-related ethos that society adopts. Ecological models clarify that harm can result from acts of commission and omission occurring at the genetic, not just gross, level. In this commentary we present examples of harm reduction from the public health genetics literature that touch on positive actions which may be taken to promote primary, secondary, and tertiary disease prevention. The avoidance of neural tube defects through cereal fortification, dietary prevention of newborn metabolic defects, and genetic testing to avoid pernicious spread of hereditary breast and ovarian cancer occupy these categories of harm reduction, each touching on starkly visible harms that could take place without proper public health efforts. Neighborhoods in low income areas in multiple countries present challenging conditions. Poor nutritional food availability and the possibility of environmental contaminants, lead being a widespread example, require attention to avoid exposure in one generation resulting in harm to the next. Genetic research has uncovered the epigenetic mechanisms behind the gene-environment interactions that may result. The solutions are both biological and social, with community resources playing a part. The unique contribution of public health genetics to the field of harm reduction is the awareness it has raised of the distinction between genotypic and phenotypic prevention, especially in the realm of prenatal genetic testing. This distinction has impacted the United States more so than other countries in terms of the range of services offered by public health authorities, and has helped to avoid labeling and stigmatization that might otherwise occur through the prevention of human characteristics. An educated public health workforce can maximize the benefits of genetic policies for physical harm reduction while minimizing the use of interventions that could otherwise result in social harm.

**Keywords:** Genetics, harm, public health, prevention, genetic testing, prenatal testing, newborn screening, neural tube defects, lead exposure, diabetes, epigenetics, inborn errors of metabolism, hemoglobinopathies, breast cancer, stigmatization, discrimination, disability rights perspective, health policy

## Introduction – Harm from the Outside-In

Harm reduction in the public health context is often thought of in the physical sense, leading to needle exchange and substance abuse prevention programs, avoidance of drunk driving, promotion of safe sex, and attention to workplace hazards. In its broadest sense, harm can entail both physical and psychosocial injury or damage. The effects of repeat discrimination can impact health. Public health authorities have coined the term “John Henryism” for the chronic disease accompanying stress and overexertion experienced by members of marginalized minority groups [1]. The legendary John Henry, for all his efforts at escaping the southern sharecropping system to win freedom, suffered considerable harm from his exertions in the form of early arthritis, peptic ulcer, and the sequelae of high blood pressure.

Harm can result from acts of commission (injurious actions, as experienced in John Henry’s time and in occupational settings today, as well as through risky behaviors) and omission (lack of attention to disease and injury as it ensues). Public health’s main focus is prevention, adopting a pro-active stance to the avoidance of harm. Preventive action can take place at a number of levels.

The Institute of Medicine has publicized a circular model of the determinants of population health which depicts the biological determinants of health centrally, community factors midway, and broad social policies at the state and national levels outermost [2]. The model is ecological in the sense that it takes into account the surrounding behavioral and social milieu. If attention is devoted to biological factors, then genes and genetic predispositions would be at the center of the circular model [3]. Public health is able to advocate for and implement action at the various levels needed to curtail harm, social and biological, gross and molecular. The field of public health genetics is aimed at the most intimate causative mechanisms underlying harm, with the goal of preventing harm at the earliest stages.

## PRIMARY PREVENTION OF HARM

The prenatal period is an especially delicate time for the developing fetus. Physical abnormalities such as placenta previa (low placement of the placenta in the womb), premature separation of the placenta, and prolapse of the umbilical cord may result in fetal hypoxia and short-term neurological deficits in the newborn, but can also result in cerebral palsy and mental retardation [4]. The harm from delayed attention to these occurrences is clear-cut; each of these maladies, further, may be caught in time with appropriate medical attention. Such events happen on an individual basis -- it is the individual family, mother, and child-to-be that benefit from the attention of the health care provider. Outcomes are not entirely predictable; the child is drawn into a family system where resources and care take center stage and provide stability.

The focus of public health providers is more population-oriented, yet it is equally concerned with the harms that may arise during the critical time before and after birth. In a review of nineteen state genetics plans, the three most common genetic programs covered birth defects, newborn screening, and childhood and adult genetic conditions such as sickle cell disease [5]. Action to avoid birth defects constitutes primary prevention (before the disease has occurred), while newborn screening and follow-up constitute secondary prevention (early in disease manifestation). It has been estimated that less than 10% of disability is due to birth defects having congenital causes that cannot easily be foreseen or managed [6]. Neural tube defects (NTD) can be prevented, however, by proper maternal folate intake. Meta-analysis suggests that folic acid fortification of food staples could prevent ~46% of NTD incidence and mortality, and ~13% of neonatal deaths due to visible congenital anomalies in the third world [7]. Public health genetics programs in the United States sponsor on their own and in partnership with the March of Dimes campaigns to promote the use of folate, particularly for women contemplating having a child. State public health programs provide teratogen information services to help pregnant mothers be alert to substances in the home or workplace environments that may pose a risk to fetal growth and development. State health departments also conduct active and passive surveillance systems to monitor birth defects.

Subtler harms with more chronic and less physically overt consequences can also occur prenatally. Diabetes during pregnancy can increase the passage of glucose across the placenta, and result in excess weight gain and metabolic abnormalities in the offspring, posing risk across generations [8]. Lead contamination reaching the fetus may result in cognitive delays in childhood [9]. Maternal diabetes can have purely intrinsic causes, such as gestational diabetes, but it can also pre-exist the period of pregnancy and be perpetuated by neighborhood and cultural dietary practices and local food availability. Diabetes associated with the food deficits in the household and neighboring environment, and lead exposure from paint and automobile proximity from previously lead-laden gasoline are public health concerns in that they can impact the wider community, thus calling for prevention measures. Both have epigenetic effects that can befall socio-economic and racial-ethnic groups differently, and carry an impact across multiple generations.

Epigenetic effects occur when environmentally induced and developmentally regulated variations are transmitted to subsequent generations of cells or organisms. They represent a form of gene-environment interaction that modifies gene operation rather than genes themselves. The literature emphasizes four main types of mechanisms: chromatin marking (e.g., methyl groups that attach to DNA, histone protein wrapping – the scaffolding of DNA), structural inheritance (mostly lower organisms), RNA-mediated inheritance, and feedback loops (gene products acting as regulators). The various measures of lead exposure, methylation of cord blood DNA and maternal tibia lead [9], are proxies for the epigenetic programming taking place in DNA at the neural level from three weeks after conception through juvenile life. Disruption of proteins that bind to methylated DNA sequences and mediate repression of gene expression has been found to alter neuronal survival, differentiation, and synaptic function [10]. DNA methylation also plays a role in downregulating the pluripotency genes in embryonic stem cells during neural induction. Lead's impact starts with maternal exposure, but continues at the cellular, anatomic, and behavioral levels in the child-to-be.

In the case of diabetes, researchers have found that maternal "overnutrition" may lead to metabolic imprinting and alteration of genes involved in the regulation of energy homeostasis. Several such sites can be influenced by DNA methylation and histone modification: leptin, *SOCS3*, and glucose transporter genes [11]. In animal studies, phenotypic (visible) and epigenetic changes can persist for at least two generations [12].

Solutions, because these conditions are so environmentally-attuned, are both biological-physiological and social, touching on community resources. Community leaders can initiate programs that make healthy foods available to neighborhoods. Community groups can decide on the wisdom of environmental hazard abatement versus avoidance policies, and can advocate for environmental justice [13].

## SECONDARY PREVENTION OF HARM

Interventions focusing on prevention of harm are the bread and butter of public health. If risk conditions can be attended to before harm occurs, then health can be preserved before it suffers substantial compromise, and the possibility exists that many at-risk people can be reached. In many situations, however, the setting has already begun to exert a health impact. An adolescent has already been exposed to substances of abuse as a result of peer pressure. A youngster has frolicked through neighborhood grounds high in lead before the possibility of lead hazard has entered people's minds. A family health history or thorough maternal history is not taken; a child in the first few days of life is born with a metabolic condition first detected in a newborn blood spot [14]. Since secondary prevention implies that harm has already begun to occur, amelioration of the condition is all the more pressing. The inborn errors of metabolism can have dire mental and physical consequences if not attended to quickly (Table 1).

The vast majority of states also screen newborns for hemoglobinopathies (sickle cell anemia, beta-thalassemia) and cystic fibrosis. These conditions are conceptually distinct from those in Table 1 in that they may have a chronic impact, but current therapies, including for beta-thalassemia, are yielding almost normal life expectancies. Worldwide, carrier and prenatal screening can lead to a reduction in the birth prevalence of thalassemia of over 90% [20], an incredible statistic considering that beta-thalassemia can take the life of children before the age of three.

**Table 1. Physical consequences of inborn errors of metabolism**

| Condition | Sequelae [15] | Interventions |
|---|---|---|
| Organic acid metabolism defects,<br>Urea acid defects | life-threatening encephalopathy, coma | dietary restriction, removal of toxic metabolites, enhancement of enzyme activity [16] |
| Biotinidase deficiency | limb weakness, hearing loss, optic atrophy, seizures and coma | avoidance of egg whites, biotin supplementation [17] |
| Galactosemia | poor weight gain, liver dysfunction, cataract formation | restriction of galactose intake, lactose-free formulas, calcium and vitamin intake [18] |
| Mucopolysachharidosis type I | mental retardation, course facial features, cardiomyopathy, hepatosplenomegaly | enzyme replacement therapy, blood stem cell transplantation [19] |

Controversy exists in the application of prenatal testing to genetic conditions that leave a relatively normal life expectancy and fairly high quality of life. Sickle cell anemia, cystic fibrosis, Down syndrome, and congenital deafness fall in this territory. Juengst and Khoury draw a distinction between "phenotypic prevention," which emphasizes efforts to prevent clinical manifestations of a genetic condition, and "genotypic prevention," bent on preventing transmission of particular genotypes to the next generation [21, 22]. The perspective of the disability community lies heavily against prenatal testing, with its abortion option [23]. States Adrienne Asch, "Autobiographical writings and family narratives testify eloquently to the rich lives and the even richer futures that are possible for people with disabilities today" [24]. The additional option of preimplantation genetic diagnosis (PGD), prenatal testing at the four- to eight-cell stage post-conception, only complicates the matter, especially considering the technology may be used to select heterozygote embryos that have only one affected gene, not two. Ethical relativism plays a part in the judgment of the technologic alternatives. The prevalence of hemoglobinopathies in diverse ethnic communities will have a different moral weight in the United Kingdom than in Germany, where eugenics remains a stark memory.

Concerns over stigmatization and discrimination persist for prospective partners who test positive for having a future at-risk child, parents who opt to give birth to a child affected with a genetic condition in the face of positive carrier and/or prenatal testing, and the child as he or she matures and applies for health insurance and employment. For example, identified carriers in a sickle cell screening program in Ochemenos, Greece were socially ostracized as being undesirable marriage partners [25]. The possibility of stigmatization in a variety of settings represents a distinct form of harm – social, not physical – and can be equally paralyzing. When an individual is discriminated against in the community or in the workplace, the harm inflicted is of a psychosocial kind, but it can compare to physical harm and have lasting repercussions. Dor Yeshorim was started in Brooklyn to protect genetic privacy, and the Americans with Disabilities Act and Genetic Information Nondiscrimination Act were legislated to guard against genetic discrimination.

Novel situations arise which move into vaster policy domains, while resurrecting memories of past discrimination. Following the 2006 death of Bennie Abram, a Rice University student-athlete, the National Collegiate Athletic Association instituted a policy of mandatory screening (can utilize former newborn screening records) to establish the sickle cell status of college athletes. The policy has stirred controversy, as its impact can be both protective and labeling – for athlete and family [26]. The American Society of Hematology has called for universal preventive interventions instead of genetic screening, a move that would avoid labeling of individuals and groups. According to a 2010 American Public Health Association policy statement on genetic and genomic literacy, these qualities are to be viewed as a capacity to see the individual at-risk not in isolation, but in the context of a social environment that provides effective resources, rights, and freedoms [27]. Public health practitioners need to be educated not just in the technical aspects of assessing potential for harm, but also the socio-ethical risks posed by various measures. Balancing must occur so that future genetic policies protect against physical harm while not inflicting social harm.

## TERTIARY PREVENTION OF HARM

The bar for implementing multi-pronged strategies to avoid harm from hereditary conditions and genetic interventions should be set high when those efforts are directed at entire populations. Caution is called for when the interventions themselves carry the possibility of harm.

Mortality from breast cancer is about 21 persons per 100,000 individuals per year. Cohort studies and clinical trials have estimated a 90% reduction in risk for hereditary breast cancer from prophylactic mastectomy, and a 49% reduction in breast cancer risk with tamoxifen treatment [28]. Oophorectomy results in comparable (80-90%) reductions in risk for ovarian cancer. Harm can be gauged in terms of the disfigurement and mortality risk from advanced breast cancer versus the psychosocial impact and disfigurement of breast removal in the case of mastectomy.

The Evaluation of Genomic Applications in Practice and Prevention (EGAPP) Working Group has moved cautiously on the relative prognostic capabilities of two tumor gene expression profiling assays that predict outcome, *MammaPrint* and *Oncotype Dx*, until further clinical trials are completed [29]. The United States Centers for Disease Control and Prevention places gene expression profiling for breast cancer in the Tier-2 category for levels of evidence [30]. Tier-1 genetic applications include those with sufficient evidence of validity and clinical utility for the test to be implemented into practice; tier-2 include those with sufficient evidence of validity and promising evidence of utility, but as yet insufficient to support a consistent recommendation for use [31]. The public health perspective is that family history of hereditary breast and ovarian cancer has sufficient evidence for referral for BRCA genetic counseling and testing (primary prevention) [32], but that secondary and tertiary prevention (where disease has already occurred) using genetic assays as prognostic indicators requires further evidence [30]. A strong level of evidence is required when moving genetic technologies to the population level for tertiary prevention.

## Conclusion – Harm in the Genetic Domain Can Be Both Physical and Social

Public health has a natural tendency to view early prevention of harm as preferable to prevention of harm that has already begun. This orientation is just as true in the realm of genetics as it is in other areas such as harm from drug abuse and injury. Because genetic identity is so tied-up with personal identity, harm from labeling individuals and groups is also a foremost consideration. Disease conditions can harm, but so can health technologies. The eugenics of the earlier part of the 20$^{th}$ Century, sickle cell screening of the 1970s, and recent encounters with pharmacotherapies targeting specific racial-ethnic groups make it paramount that the definition of harm including genetics be extrapolated through a lens of physical and social harm. Public health genetics has developed a code of evidence – Tier 1 through Tier 3 applications – that assists in deciphering when a genetic technology will cause the least harm while offering the greatest benefit. This system respects the *primum non nocere* – "first, do no harm" – principle as primary in the health field.

As Pernick has stated, the degree of advancement in genetics is no antidote to the possibility that the use of a given technology will not have socially untoward effects [33]. Transparency is required so that a stiff view is taken before policies are solidified and the technology becomes mainstream. Given proper cautions, we hope to have established that public health has much to say and recommend about interventions applied to the most central level of harm, that occurring at the molecular genetic level. Overarching conceptual frameworks dealing with levels of prevention and degrees of evidence have just as much applicability in the field of genetics as they do in other public health arenas that forecast and avoid harm. In this light, much can be done to secure the safety of the youngest among us, born into the world in such a fragile state, as well as those of us who have been weathered by time, with our disease susceptibilities exposed. Harm, like one's genetic fate, is not written in stone. The health practitioner and consumer have the power to prevent harm in an equitable way, allowing the effect to transcend the single individual and spread to the wider population.

## REFERENCES


[1] James, S. B. John Henryism and the health of African-Americans. *Culture Med. Psychiatry* 1994; 18(2): 163-182.

[2] Institute of Medicine. *The future of the public's health in the 21st century*. Committee on Assuring the Health of the Public in the 21st Century. Board on Health Promotion and Disease Prevention. Washington, D.C.: The National Academies Press; 2003.

[3] Modell, S. M., Kardia, S. L. R., Citrin, T., King, S. B. The ecological model in genetics and religion. In: G. Simpson and S. Payne, eds. *Religion and ethics*. Hauppauge, NY: Nova Science Publishers; 2013, pp. 99-121.

[4] Page, E. W., Villee, C. A., Villee, D. B. *Human reproduction: the core content of obstetrics, gynecology and perinatal medicine*. 2nd ed. Philadelphia: W.B. Saunders Company; 1976.

[5] Wang, G., Watts, C. The role of genetics in the provision of essential public health services. *Am. J. Public Health* 2007; 97(4): 620-625.

[6] Kullman, K. Genetic risks: the implications of embryo screening. *Spiegel* Aug. 2, 2013: 3. www.spiegel.de/international/germany/controversial-pid-embryo-screening-in-germany-a-882067.html.

[7] Blencowe, H., Cousens, S., Modell, B., Lawn, J. Folic acid to reduce neonatal mortality from neural tube disorders. *Int. J. Epidemiol.* 2010; 39 Suppl. 1: i110-i121.

[8] Kuzawa, C. W., Sweet, E. Epigenetics and the embodiment of race: developmental origins of US racial disparities in cardiovascular health. *Am. J. Hum. Biol.* 2009; 21(1): 2-15.

[9] Pilsner, J. R., Hu, H., Ettinger, A., Sanchez, B. N., Wright, R. O., Cantonwine, D., Lazarus, A., Lamadrid-Figueroa, H., Maercado-Garcia, A., Tellez-Rojo, M. M., Hernandez-Avila, M. Influence of prenatal lead exposure on genomic methylation of cord blood DNA. *Environ. Health Perspect.* 2009; 117(9): 1466-77.

[10] Senut, M.-C., Cingolani, P., Sen, A., Kruger, A., Shaik, A., Hirsch, H., Suhr, S. T., Ruden, D. Epigenetics of early-life lead exposure and effects on brain development. *Epigenomics* 2012; 4(6): 665-674.

[11] Dabelea, D., Crume, T. Maternal environment and the transgenerational cycle of obesity and diabetes. *Diabetes* 2011; 60(7): 1849-55.

[12] Gluckman, P. D., Hanson, M. A., Buklijas, T., Low, F. M., Beedle, A. S. Epigenetic mechanisms that underpin metabolic and cardiovascular diseases. *Nat. Rev. Endocrinol.* 2009; 5(7): 401-408.

[13] Sze, J., Prakash, S. Human genetics, environment, and communities of color: ethical and social implications. *Environ. Health Perspect.* 2004; 112(6): 740-745.

[14] Khoury, M. J. and the Genetics Working Group. From genes to public health: the applications of genetic technology in disease prevention. *Am. J. Public Health* 1996; 86(12): 1717-22.

[15] Burton, B. K. Inborn errors of metabolism in infancy: a guide to diagnosis. *Pediatrics* 1998; 102(6): E69.

[16] Seashore, M. R. The organic acidemias: an overview. *GeneReviews* 2009. www.ncbi.nlm.nih.gov/books/NBK1134.

[17] Wolf, B. Biotinidase deficiency. *GeneReviews* 2013. www.ncbi.nlm.nih.gov/books/NBK1322.

[18] Berry, G. T. Classic galactosemia and clinical variant galactosemia. *GeneReviews* 2014. www.ncbi.nlm.nih.gov/books/NBK1518.

[19] Clarke, L. A., Heppner, J. Mucopolysaccharidosis type I. *GeneReviews* 2011. www.ncbi.nlm.nih.gov/books/NBK1162.

[20] Modell, B., Darlison, M. Global epidemiology of haemoglobin disorders and derived service indicators. *Bull. World Health Organ.* 2008; 85(6): 480-487.

[21] Juengst, E. T. "Prevention" and the goals of genetic medicine. *Hum. Gene Ther.* 1995; 6(12): 1595-605.

[22] Khoury, M. J. Genetic epidemiology and the future of disease prevention and public health. *Epidemiol. Rev.* 1997; 19(1); 175-180.

[23] Koch, T. Disability and difference: balancing social and physical constructions. *J. Med. Ethics* 2001; 27(6): 370-376.

[24] Asch, A. Prenatal diagnosis and selective abortion: a challenge to practice and policy. *Am. J. Public Health* 1999; 89(11): 1649-57.

[25] Wilfond, B. S., Fost, N. The cystic fibrosis gene: medical and social implications for heterozygote detection. *J. Am. Med. Assoc.* 1990; 263 (10): 2777-83.

[26] Bonham, V. L., Dover, G. J., Brody, L. C. Screening student athletes for sickle cell trait – a social and clinical experiment. *N. Engl. J. Med.* 2010; 363 (11): 997-999.

[27] American Public Health Association. *Strengthening genetic and genomic literacy. Policy No. 201012.* Nov. 2010. www.apha.org/policies-and-advocacy/public-health-policy-statements/policy-database/2014/07/30/16/37/strengthening-genetic-and-genomic-literacy.

[28] Petrucelli, N., Daly, M. B., Feldman, G. L. Hereditary breast and ovarian cancer due to mutations in *BRCA1* and *BRCA2*. *Genet. Med.* 2010; 12 (5): 245-259.

[29] Evaluation of Genomic Applications in Practice and Prevention (EGAPP) Working Group. Recommendations from the EGAPP Working Group: can tumor gene expression profiling improve outcomes in patients with breast cancer? *Genet. Med.* 2009; 11(1): 66-73.

[30] Centers for Disease Control and Prevention, Office of Public Health Genomics. *Genomic tests and family history by levels of evidence: tier 2.* Atlanta, GA. 2014. www.cdc.gov/genomics/gtesting/tier2.htm.

[31] Khoury, M. J., Bowen, M. S., Burke, W., Coates, R. J., Dowling, N. F., Evans, J. P., Reyes, M., St. Pierre, J. Current priorities for public health practice in addressing the role of human genomics in improving population health. *Am. J. Prev. Med.* 2011; 40(4): 486-493.

[32] Centers for Disease Control and Prevention, Office of Public Health Genomics. *Genomic tests and family history by levels of evidence: tier 1*. Atlanta, GA. 2014. www.cdc.gov/genomics/gtesting/tier.htm.

[33] Pernick, M. S. Eugenics and public health in American history. *Am. J. Public Health* 1997; 87(11): 1767-72.

In: Public Health and Harm Reduction
Editor: Meredith B. Morris

ISBN: 978-1-63482-159-9


*Chapter 3*

# ENDOCRINE DISRUPTORS, OBESITY AND PUBLIC HEALTH: PERSPECTIVES ON HARM REDUCTION

***Minelli Salles Alves Fernandes[1], Melvy Marin Rivero[1], Marcela Miranda Salles[3], Denise Rosso Tenório Wanderley Rocha[1,2] and Alberto Krayyem Arbex[1,2*]***

[1]Endocrinology Department, Medical Institute for Teaching and Research—IPEMED, Brazil
[2]Federal University of Rio de Janeiro, Brazil
[3]Pharmacy College, Federal University of Bahia, Brazil

## ABSTRACT

Endocrine-disrupting Chemicals (EDCs) are exogenous chemicals that interfere with the metabolism and action of various hormones and intracellular signaling. The interference in the differentiation of adipocytes and weight homeostasis are key actions of EDCs, which could possibly be associated with obesity. EDCs may also have effects during intrauterine development, contributing to increase an individual's weight

---

* Corresponding author: Prof. Alberto K. Arbex, IPEMED BRAZIL, Praça Vereador Rocha Leão, 10–Copacabana, Cep 22.031-060, Rio de Janeiro–RJ, BRAZIL. Email: albertoarbex @gmail.com.

in adulthood. Obesity is a pandemic nowadays, increasing especially among children, and also in developing countries. It is a chronic inflammatory multifactorial disease. Current studies suggest a possible association with pre or postnatal exposure to endocrine disruptors. These 'obesogenic' disruptors are found in food packaging, cosmetics, industrial waste, organochlorine pesticides and fuels. The most common contaminants are Bisphenol A (BPA), phthalates, phytoestrogens, dioxine and DDT. Despite the correlation between increased body mass and adipogenesis by the action of EDCs, their molecular mechanisms remain poorly understood. These substances affect the endocrine function by stimulating PPARy receptors or acting as antiandrogens - aromatase inhibitors, resulting in increased lipogenesis. Those receptors are associated the differentiation, activation and maturation of adipocytes in fat synthesis in cells. They can also act on nuclear receptors and on the nervous system. Several factors such as age and length of exposure can influence the effect of EDCs, but the dose-response relationship remains unclear. The goal of this chapter is to develop a critical review of the literature on the influence of environmental contaminants in the development of adiposity.

**Keywords:** Endocrine disruptors, environmental exposure, lipogenesis, obesity, public health

# 1. Introduction

Obesity is a chronic and multifactorial disease, defined as a body mass index (BMI) greater than or equal to 30.0 $kg/m^2$, whose prevalence has reached alarming numbers worldwide [1,2]. Data from the World Health Organization (WHO) shows that 1.6 billion people are overweight and 400 million are obese. It seems that by 2015, these values shall reach 3.3 billion and 700 million, respectively [3]. In Brazil, the proportion of people who are overweight increased from 42.7% in 2006 to 48.5% in 2011, while the percentage of obese rose from 11.4 to 15.8% during the same period [4].

Obesity is associated with high morbidity and mortality. It favors the occurrence of various morbidities, such as type 2 diabetes mellitus (T2DM), dyslipidemia, hypertension, cardiovascular diseases, degenerative joint disease, various types of cancer (breast, liver, colon, cervix, prostate, etc.), sleep apnea, among others [5].

It involves causal factors such as energy imbalance, genetic predisposition, environmental and cultural factors. These are usually related to a sedentary lifestyle and poor dietary habits, such as an increased caloric intake. However, other reasons may be associated with obesity: sleep deprivation, pregnancy later in life, intrauterine factors, use of medications such as antidepressants, low calcium intake, some viruses and bacteria, and endocrine-disrupting chemicals, or simply 'Endocrine Disruptors' (here refered to as 'EDCs') [3].

An Endocrine Disruptor is defined as an exogenous substance or mixture in the environment that alters the function of the endocrine system, causing adverse health effects in an intact organism, or in its progeny [6].

It is reported that EDCs affect the endocrine function, since it can stimulate PPARγ receptors and retinoid X receptors (RXRs), acting as anti-androgens or as aromatase inhibitors, resulting in increased lipogenesis. Both receptors are related to the differentiation, maturation and activation in synthesis of fat cells adipocytes. They can also act on other nuclear receptors and nervous system [3].

There is a variety of endocrine disruptors in the environment. Regarding obesity, it is believed that its primary action relates to the interference in the adipocyte differentiation and homeostasis mechanisms of weight, the most widely substance studied beying 'Bisphenol A' (BPA) [7]

In Brazil, the highest prevalences of obesity is found in the most industrialized regions of the country as in the southern region, therefore where potentially greater public exposure to EDCs occurs [8].

This chapter aims to bring relevant information about the most relevant EDCs, their probable mechanisms involved and occurrence in the environment, focusing on participation in these metabolic disorders possibly involved in the pathogenesis of obesity.

## 2. THE ENDOCRINE SYSTEM

Among the various systems that build the human physiology, the endocrine system is essential for life maintenance. It consists of a set of glands located in different areas of the body, such as the thyroid, gonads and adrenal glands, and the hormones synthesized by them, such as thyroxin, estrogen and progesterone, testosterone and adrenaline [9].

Hormones are chemicals (messengers) produced and secreted by the endocrine glands and that, released into the bloodstream, coordinate the functioning of the organism as a whole. Some functions they control are: whole organs activities, levels of salts, sugars and liquid in the blood, energy use and storage, growth and development of a particular organism, its reproduction, their sexual characteristics, etc.[10]

To perform their natural actions, the hormones must have affinity and specificity to receptors located in the membrane, cytoplasm or nucleus of cells. These proteic receptors undergo conformational changes after hormone binding and thereby initiate the metabolic reactions on target cells. The receivers are not fixed components, and may vary as to its location and numeric distribution for each tissue and consequently varying the intensity of the response [9].

The hormonal action occurs from two basic mechanisms: activation of receptors on the cell membrane and intranuclear activation. There are four types of membrane receptors and nuclear receptors of both types. The nuclear type 1 receptor binds to steroids (estrogen, androgen, progesterone, glucocorticoids and mineralocorticoid) and type 2 binds to thyroid hormones, vitamin D, retinoic acid, free fatty acids and eicosanoids. The latter has several natural receptor ligands, and the PPARγ of them, and molecular target of several endocrine disruptors [11].

The DNA binding domains of the nuclear receptors are composed of two zinc finger containing sequences specific for the recognition of target genes. Most nuclear receptors bind to DNA as dimers and thus each monomer recognize a pattern or sequence of DNA. The type 1 receptors bind as homodimers to DNA and type 2 receptors as heterodimers in combination with retinoid X receptors (RXRs) [12].

Therefore, extremely low concentrations of a particular hormone generate and effect, producing a natural response. However, these hormone receptors may also bind to other chemicals. This explains why certain endocrine disruptors present in the body, even in very low concentrations, being able to generate an effect, therefore causing a response [10].

Abnormalities in the endocrine system occur when the exogenous interfering substance, an EDC, interacts with hormone receptors, altering its natural response. Two distinct processes can be triggered. The chemical substance can bind to the estrogen receptor, thus producing an answer, then acting as a mimic, i.e., mimicking the action of a particular hormone. This process is called 'agonist effect'. If the chemical substance binds to the receptor but no response is produced, it is acting as a blocker, or will prevent the interaction between the natural hormone and its respective receptor. This process is called 'antagonist effect' [10].

Regarding obesity, fat mass itself is determined by the balance between degradation (lipolysis) and synthesis (lipogenesis). The sympathetic nervous system is the main stimulator of lipolysis, reducing fat stores, when the energy of the individual demands is increased. When the input exceeds energy use, lipogenesis occurs in liver and adipose tissue. This is influenced by a high-carbohydrate diet and hormones (mainly leptin, insulin and growth hormone – GH) through a modification of transcription factors such as PPAR (*peroxisome proliferator-activated receptor*). The main hormone involved in fat storage is insulin, which decreases lipogenesis. PPAR transcription factor, insulin sensitizers of the thiazolidinedione affects gene transcription of many enzymes involved in the metabolism of fat and glucose, also participating in the differentiation of pre-adipocytes into mature adipocytes. The other participant hormones in the regulation of body fat reserves include testosterone, thyroid hormone and dehydroepiandrosterone [9].

One of the leading hormonal axes is the hypothalamic-pituitary-gonadal, where the obesogenic action of sexual steroids is extensively studied. Estrogens are *protective* against adult abdominal obesity and metabolic disease, whereas perinatal exposure to estrogen has the opposite effect. Rats who had their ovaries removed developed abdominal obesity, which was then reversed with estrogen treatment. Consistent with this observation, the loss of estrogen receptor alpha (ER-α) resulted in an increase in size of white adipose deposits, the central weight gain, and impaired glucose metabolism. The most common types of receptors are the ER-α and ER-β, which vary among tissues. ER-α are found mainly in the breast and uterus and ER-β, bone and cardiovascular system [13].

PPARs are receptors that play a critical role in lipid metabolism and adipogenesis. PPAR-gamma is described as a regulator of fat in the development of master cell with the activation necessary for the differentiation and maturation of adipocytes. The organotins, one of the environmental contaminants, inappropriately activates these receptors, stimulating the differentiation of adipocytes, thus contributing to susceptibility to obesity and metabolic disorders [14].

EDCs are absorbed dermally, nasally or orally, and begin to interfere with the balance of the endocrine system, breaking the natural sequence of self-regulation mechanisms.

# 3. Endocrine Disruptors

## 3.1. Definition, Properties and Occurrence

As defined by the US Environmental ProtectionAgency, **Endocrine-Disrupting Chemicals (EDCs),** also known as **Disruptors** or **Interferents** or also **Endocrine Disturbers** correspond to "*exogenous agents that interfere with the synthesis, secretion, transport, metabolism, action or elimination of one or more hormones current natural responsible for homeostasis, reproduction, development and/or behavior of organisms*" [15].

Among the numerous chemicals acting as EDCs are agrochemicals and pesticides, industrial waste plastics production of components and derivatives, dyes commonly used in the marine industry, detergents, heavy metals, drugs and phytoestrogens [16]. Each environmental contaminant category shows a specific potential for acting as a metabolic disruptor substance, according to its exposure and origin (Table 1).

Several mechanisms are proposed for these agents, but one common feature is that they are chemicals that can interfere with the endocrine system in several animal species, including humans and their descendants. Such substances can be by anthropic nature or called xenoestrogenic, which means that they may be produced or not by the human body, and may also be of natural origin, such as for example, phytoestrogens [10].

Synthetic anabolic agents – also named xenoestrogens - are used in animal feed, in cosmetics and medicines (Diethylstilbestrol), as solvents and industrial lubricants (Dioxins, Polychlorinated Biphenyls and Polybrominated Biphenyls), plasticizers (phthalates and Bisphenol A) and organic pollutants POPs-persistent (metoxychlorine, DDT, Toxaphene) [12, 17].

Due to its chemical properties of stability, toxicity and lipid solubility, many of these chemicals, even if mankind interrupts its current production, will still remain for several years in the environment [18]. These substances are found in the soil and at sediments of rivers, and are easily transported from the atmosphere or from their sources over long distances. They accumulate along the trophic chain, representing a serious threat to the health of all organisms involved and especially to humans [19].

EDCs present as organic or inorganic substances. They are present in developed regions through the production of waste and industrial by-products and their effluents, in addition to large deposits and landfills that are responsible for the contamination of soil, groundwater and water sources for public supply. In rural areas, EDCs are found in agricultural products, such as pesticides and fungicides of different classes (for example: organochlorines, carbamates, pyrethrins and others) [19].

Humans and animals are exposed to the EDCs by different ways, such as food and water intake, inhaling dust and gases or even through the skin. They may also overcome the placenta, being transported from the mother to the fetus, and traces of these compounds or mixtures have in fact been detected in breast milk [19].

**Table 1. Origin and forms of occurrence of the main agents with potential for ED**

| Origin | Use and Occurrence | Chemicals Representatives |
|---|---|---|
| Incinerators and Sanitary Landfill | Municipal Waste Incineration, Industrial Waste and Hospital Equipment | Dioxin, Dibenzo-p-Dioxins Polychlorinated and Dibenzofurans Polychlorinated (PCBs) |
| Pesticides Organochlorine | Crops and Creations Animals and Still Fighting Malaria Mosquito Vector | DDT, Dieldrin, Aldrin, Toxaphene, Lindane |
| Herbicides | Agricultural Growing | Alachlor, Atrazine, Permethrin and Trifluralin |
| Ports and Marine Industry | Protective Paint Used to Cover the Hull of Navigations | Tributyltin (TBT) |
| Water Treatment Network | Flocculant Water Treatment and Sewage | Acrylamide |
| Industrial Wastewater | Alkylphenols Used as Surfactants Agents in Oil Removal | Nonylphenol |
| Petrochemical Industry | Tar, Asphalt, Diesel Emission, Coke Ovens, Grease and Mineral Oils | Benzopyrene and Benzoantracene |
| Plastic Production and Epoxi Resin | Plastic Polycarbonates And Food Cans Jacket | Bisphenol-A |
| Industrial Wastewater | Plasticizers, Varnish, Cosmetics | Phthalates (Dibutyl-Phthalate and Butylbenzyl-Phthalate) |
| Synthetic Hormones | Drugs and Animals Anabolic Drugs Present in Meat | 17-b-Estradiol, Estrone, Testosterone E Ethinyl-Estradiol |
| Phytoestrogens | Formula from Soybean | Genistein, Daidzein, Lignans E Coumestrol |

### 3.2. Mechanisms of Action

As long as they belong to different categories, there is no single mechanism of action applied to EDCs. Its effects depend directly on the route of exposure, dose, duration of contact and toxicological principles of the disruptor analised.

Endocrine disruptors may be classified according to the hormonal category of function that is affected. Most display steroid function, affecting the action of sex hormones such as testosterone and estrogen; but there are also those that disrupt thyroid function, mimicking or blocking triiodothyronine (T3) and thyroxine (T4), and some act disturbing prolactin and GH (growth hormone) homeostasis [20].

EDCs act mimicking (agonists) or blocking (antagonist) the action of certain hormones by binding to specific intranuclear receptors or in cell membrane [10]. Other pathways can also be activated by signaling through EDCs, such as neurotransmitter receptors (dopamine receptor, serotonin and norepinephrine) and orphan receptors (Aryl-hydrocarbon receptor- AhR), and enzymatic pathways involved in the biosynthesis and/or hormone metabolism [17].

The main effect is observed in estrogen pathways, binding to estrogen receptors, where EDCs may block the aromatase enzyme, which is involved in the balance of estrogen and androgen synthesis, commonly seen after the exposure to some pesticides and Tributiline compounds. The hormone transportation process can also be used to target certain disruptors which bind to active sites of protein ligand carriers competing with the endogenous hormones, thus affecting its distribution [21,22].

EDCs have genomic and non genomic actions, according to the binding site and the changes induced in the affected cell. Through the genomic intranuclear pathway, the binding of a disruptor agent to the Estrogen Receptor may lead to a conformational change of it. This structural change favors the stabilization and increased affinity of the receptor-ligand complex, which will then act on the DNA strand as a transcriptional factor, and recruit other activatiors/repressors that together regulate the synthesis of specific proteins [21].

The estrogen agonist or antagonist action varies according to the properties of endocrine disruptor and also with the tissue where the receptors are expressed. There are disruptors that act as androgens, competing with dihydrotestosterone for same receiver.

In summary, EDCs might interfere with the endocrine system in at least three ways: 1) by mimicking the action of an endogenous hormone like estrogen and testosterone; 2) blocking the receptors in cells specific for those hormones, preventing their action; and finally 3) affecting the synthesis, transport, metabolism, distribution and excretion of hormones and/or neurotransmitters [10].

## 3.3. Endocrine Disruptors in Human Health

Scientific evidence shows that some congenital abnormalities in animals and humans may be caused by endocrine disruptors present in the environment such as insecticides, fungicides, herbicides, heavy metals, organic chemical solvents like PCBs and polychlorinated biphenyls, drugs and phytoestrogens [23].

Some of these endocrine disruptors alter the steroidal hormones and may cause damage to sexual differentiation, with the consequent masculinization and feminization and even infertility [20].

These compounds are characterized by mimicking the structure and function of natural sex steroids, leading to endocrine disorders that may result in abnormal sexual and reproductive function in animals and humans [24]. Among the reproductive abnormalities observed in males are hypospadias, cryptorchidism and decrease in semen quality, which together form the so-called 'Dysgenic Testicular Syndrome' [25].

Urogenital hypospadias have been associated with imbalance and hormonal changes during pregnancy. Fetuses might be naturally exposed to major hormonal fluctuations (estrogen and progesterone) that can be determining factors in uretral closure and testicular position the child [26]. Chemicals disrupting the pituitary-gonadal axis can cause genetic mutations in the fetus and change the state of methylation and demethylation in specific genes that may impact postnatal life. This impact is observed in the reduction of sperm count and motility in semen, infertility and even the increased incidence of testicular cancer in adulthood [25].

In addition to the ability of crossing barriers and bioaccumulate, EDCs exert *transgenerational* effect, which means they can cause changes throughout adult life of the individual, reaching also his offspring. This is explained by epigenetic mutational action in the DNA of cells, which will perpetuate it abnormally during the process of cell division. This poses a serious threat to future generations [30].

Regarded as a highly harmful substance to human health, a strong example is the Diethylstillbestrol (DES), a potent synthetic estrogen commonly used between the years 1940 to 1970 to prevent miscarriages by progesterone deficiency, and in late stages of pregnancy to prevent premature births and placental hemorrhage [27].

Studies showed that as a result of hormone-disrupting and carcinogenicity, women who therapeutically used DES during pregnancy, had more cases of breast cancer after 30 years from exposure. The effects of this disruptor act via placenta during pregnancy, and cause serious reproductive complications in adult life of these sons and daughters. Abnormalities such as endometriosis, uterine malformations, paraovarian cysts, many organ disorders of the reproductive system, benign vaginal adenosis and uterine myomas are noticed in the offspring of mothers exposed to DES in pregnancy [24,27].

Regarding the carcinogenic potential of EDCs, the neoplastic effect vary according to some relevant factors, such as: the degree of sexual maturation of the individual, dose, time and extension of exposure to the substance. Neoplasms such as vaginal adenosis, breast cancer, testicular and prostate cancer may be caused by EDCs as the Bisphenol A (BPA), Diethylstilbestrol and dioxins [28].

Besides their action on the reproductive system, there are studies that show the participation of EDCs in thyroid dysfunction, thus indirectly affecting the functioning of memory and human behavior [31, 32].

The risk is posed because any stage of the complex physiological thyroid system may be affected, ranging from the iodine uptake, the production of thyroid hormone, interconversion between T3 to T4, cellular uptake, activation of receptors and up to the degradation or elimination of these hormones [29].

Thyroid disruptors correspond to subtypes of EDCs that interfere either with the function of the thyroid gland or directly in the hypothalamus-pituitary-thyroid axis and in their hormone receptors. This action causes changes in the development and glandular functioning, varying according to the individual's stage of development during the exposure [31].

Among the key players as thyroid disruptors are the polychlorinated biphenyls (PCBs), BPA, p-dioxin-tetrachlorodibenzen (TCDD), poly-chlorinated-dibenzoflurane, perchlorate, pentachlorophenol, triclosan, poly-brominated diphenyl, and also synthetic chemical compounds present in plastics, detergents and flame retardants and thiocyanate But there are also isoflavones, which are present in the nature. [29].

Exposure to these agents during prenatal life and early stage childhood may lead to deficits in learning, low IQ, behavioral abnormalities and mental retardation. In adults who had contact to thyroid disruptors auto-immune disorders may be diagnosed, neoplasms, clinical and subclinical hypothyroidism and increased cardiovascular risk related to altered lipid metabolism [30].

Many alterations such as increased body mass and fat content may result from prenatal exposure to EDCs in this case called obesogens such as: abnormal differentiation of adipocytes, impaired glucose homeostasis and insulin resistance. These may be caused by synthetic estrogen, genistein (isoflavone) and BPA [31].

This is how EDCs affect energy balance of the body and thus corroborate the onset of type II diabetes and/or obesity [32].

## 3.4. Endocrine Disruptors: Contribution to the Occurrence of Obesity

The obesogens are endocrine disruptors that may be present in the environment and/or in food, and inappropriately regulate lipid accumulation and adipogenesis [33].

The individual's stage of development, once more is a determining factor for the influence of obesogens in human homeostasis. There are strong evidences that the intrauterine development period is more vulnerable to the effect of promoting adipogenesis in the fetus than in adults [32]. This is explained by the absence of protective effects such as DNA repair, mature immune system, detoxifying liver enzymes in sufficient quantity and a complete blood-brain barrier, such as the one that exists in adults [33].

According to its mechanisms of action, the agonist or antagonist of growth hormone receptors, thyroid, estrogen, androgen and glucocorticoid, each obesogen may interact in different ways on the metabolic control [31].

Among the different disruptors, there are some classes of drugs that contribute to weight gain in humans, such as thiazolidinediones-oral antidiabetic drugs, tricyclic antidepressants, serotonin reuptake inhibitors and atypical antipsychotics such as olanzapine [33].

A variety of target tissues are involved in energy homeostasis, including hypothalamus and fat cells. Some obesogens can connect directly to hypothalamic neurons in the brain in the early stages of life and alter the expression of key regulators of appetite [34].

Besides neuroendocrine action, it is inferred that there is a role of estrogen and its receptors as obesity-determining in animals and humans. Estrogens in adults are protective against the accumulation of abdominal fat and metabolic syndrome, while in the prenatal stage this exposure has the opposite effect, as studies in animals showed [6].

Certain environmental agents and other stressors act during intrauterine development and may lead to obesity later in adulthood. This is why the "thrifty" phenomenon is postulated, where poor maternal nutrition, smoking, diabetes and exposure to contaminants might produce epigenetic changes (changes in the pattern of DNA methylation) that will be passed on and will lead to obesity [35].

At the molecular level, experimental evidences indicate that members of the superfamily of nuclear receptors PPAR-γ (peroxisome proliferator activated receptor) are the main target for the action, in particular for organotins and phthalates such as Tributiline (TBT) and tripheniletine commonly used in industry, plastic packaging and agriculture [17]. The same mechanism is observed for Rosiglitazone, a former drug representative of the thiazolidinedione class, no longer in use [33].

The PPAR-γ receptors are a group of nuclear receptor proteins that act as transcriptional factors to be dimerized with RXR receptors (Retinoid-X Receptor) by regulating gene expression. They are present in fat tissue, and its activation promotes adipocyte differentiation and lipogenesis [17].

The intake of isoflavones such as genistein, as part of a balanced diet, may raise questions regarding the benefits of soy. In high concentrations, genistein promotes lipogenesis through the activation of the pathway of PPAR-γ and independent estrogen receptors [17].

Another example of obesogen is Bisphenol A (BPA), which is found in increased amounts in the urine of women and men exposed to the chemical agent in the United States, and was correlated with weight gain of these individuals as measured by the BMI (body mass index) and abdominal circumference, independent of traditional risk factors (smoking, alcohol consumption, high cholesterol and other) [14]. The long-term exposure to BPA may cause hyperinsulinemia, insulin resistance and chronic predisposition for the development of type II diabetes [17].

Dioxins are polychlorinated compounds which generically refer to dibenzo-p-polychlorinated dioxins (PCDDs), polychlorinated biphenyls (PCBs) and that the designation recently appeared PSPs or Persistent Organic Pollutants to describe these compounds as a whole [36].

Due to PCB's different properties (non-flammable, chemical stability, high boiling point and electrical insulation) they were used in plastics, pigments, paper, etc. Studies demonstrate that the PCB-126 reduces androgen synthesis in a dose-dependent manner in H295R human adrenocortical and gonadal cells and at high concentrations, they stimulate the synthesis of cortisol and aldosterone by activating enzymes of cytochrome P450 (CYP11B1 and CYP11B2) which catalyze the final steps of the synthesis pathway of these steroids. Therefore, alterations of these steroidal hormones might be associated with high incidence of diabetes and cardiovascular mortality observed in highly exposed to PCBs individuals [12].

PCBs are highly resistant to degradation. They accumulate in fatty tissue, causing the exposure to occur through the consumption of fish or another predator in the food chain. Exposure to PCBs was associated with pubertal delay and decreased testicular size in boys and delayed appearance of breasts in girls [18].

## CONCLUSION

Current medical literature suggests a crucial role of endocrine disruptors in the etiology of obesity, which is not yet fully understood. The evidence points out to the action of EDCs in endocrine homeostasis disturbances. Due to the wide range of industrial chemicals to which humans are exposed, it is no longer possible to ignore its effects on the human body. Further research is necessary to elucidate all possible interactions between environmental substances and metabolic regulation changes. By understanding the effect of EDCs on the genesis or exacerbation of obesity, we might change the perception of its etiology. Obesity prevention and treatment could be changed in its essence.

Global strategies to control the harm that the endocrine disruptors represent are being constantly discussed. Creating specific guidelines for evaluating the safety of chemicals could be a way, and also a compounds risk assessment (evaluation of dose-response characterization of endocrine risk), discussion of current knowledge with legislators and regulatory agencies and finally, educate and inform the world's population about EDCs. The precautionary principle of Law should be strongly considered in this case, before we face the serious consequences of such exposure.

# References


[1] Khan A; Raza S; Khan Y; Aksoy T; Khan M; Weinberger Y; Goldman J. Current updates in the medical management of obesity. *Recent Pat Endocr Metab Immune Drug Discov.*, 2012, 6(2), 117-128.

[2] World Health Organization. Obesity – preventing and managing the global epidemic. Report of a WHO Consultation (Technical Report Series, nº. 894). Geneva, 1998.

[3] Júnior, R; Fernandes, V. Obesidade e disruptores endócrinos. Revista da ABESO. Edição nº 42 - Ano VIX - Nº 42 - Nov/2009. Disponível em: http://www.abeso.org.br/pagina/263/artigo---obesidade-e-disruptores-endocrinos.shtml. Accessed August, 2014.

[4] Brasil, Ministério da Saúde. Portal da Saúde – SUS. Disponível em: http://portalsaude.saude.gov.br/portalsaude/noticia/4718/162/quase-metade-da-populacao-brasileira-esta-acima-do-peso.html. Accessed August, 2014.

[5] Williams Textbook of Endocrinology. 12th Edition. Lippincott. 1920 p.

[6] Legler, J; Hamers, T; van der Bor MES, Schoeters G, van der Ven L, Eggesbo M, Koppe J, Feinberg M, Trnovec T. The OBELIX project: early life exposure to endocrine disruptors and obesity. *Am J Clin Nutr*, 2011, 94, 1933S-1938S.

[7] Shankar, A; Teppala, S; Sabanayagam, C. Urinary bisphenol A levels and measures of obesity: results from the national health and nutrition examination survey, 2003-2008. *Endocrinology*, 2012, 1-6.

[8] Vedana EHB, Peres MA, Neves J, Rocha GC, Longo GZ. Obesity Prevalence and Factors Potentially Causal in Adults in Southern Brazil. Arq Bras Endocrinol Metab, 2008, 52/7.

[9] Molina, PE (LANGE). Fisiologia Endócrina. 4ª ed. Editora McGrawHill, 2014.

[10] Ghiselli, G; Jardim, WF. Interferentes endócrinos no ambiente. *Quim. Nova*, 2007, 30(3), 695-706.

[11] Jameson, J. Harrison's *endocrinology* 3rd ed: New York: McGraw Hill, 2013. 560 p.

[12] Montenegro R; Fontenele EG; Martins MR; Quidute ARP. Contaminantes ambientais e interferentes endócrinos. *Arq Bras Endocrinol Metab*, 2009, 1(54), 6-16.

[13] Janesick, A; Blumberg, B. Obesogens, Stem Cells and the Developmental Programming of Obesity. *Int J Androl.*, 2012, 35(3), 437–448.

[14] Hatch EE; Nelson JW; Stahlhut RW; Webster TF. Association of endocrines disruptors and obesity: perspectives from epidemiologic studies. *Int. J. Androl*, 2010, 33(2), 324-332.

[15] U.S. Environmental Protection Agency. Special Report on Environmental Endocrine Disruption: An Effects Assessment and Analisys. Risk Assessment Forum. EPA/630/R-96/012, Washington, D.C, 1997.

[16] Sahay, RK; Nagendar, JR; Hyderabad, D. Endocrine Disruptors. In: _. (Org). *Medicine Update*, 2012, 22(6), 306-314.

[17] Kandarakis, D; et al. Endocrine-Disrupting Chemicals: An Endocrine Society Scientific Statement. *Endocrine Reviews*, 2009, 30(4), 293-342.

[18] Alves C; Flores LC; Cerqueira TS; Toralles MBP. Exposição ambiental a interferentes endócrinos com atividade estrogênica e sua associação com distúrbios puberais em crianças. Cad. Saúde Pública, Rio de Janeiro, 2007, 23(5), 1005-1014, 2007.

[19] Guimarães, JRPF. Disruptores endócrinos no meio ambiente: um problema de saúde pública e ocupacional. Associação de Combate aos POPs- Associação de Consciência à Prevenção Ocupacional, Santos, mar., 2005. Disponível em: http://www.acpo.org.br/.

[20] WHO. State of the Science of Endocrine Disrupting Chemicals, 2012. IOMC (INTER-ORGANISATION PROGRAMME FOR SOUND MANAGEMENT OF CHEMICALS). GENEVA, 2012.

[21] Moraes NV; Oliveira DP; Grando MD; Valerio DAR. Exposição ambiental a desreguladores endócrinos: alterações na homeostase dos hormônios esteroidais e tireoidianos. *Rev Bras de Toxicologia*, 2008, 21(1), 1-8.

[22] Pakdel, F; Habauzit, D; Kerdivel, G. Assessment and Molecular Actions of Endocrine- Disrupting Chemicals that Interfere with Estrogen Receptor Pathways. *International Journal of Endocrinology*, 2013, 1-14.

[23] Dezotti, M; Bila, DM. Desreguladores endócrinos no meio ambiente: efeitos e consequências. *Quím. Nova*, 2007, 30(3), 651-666.

[24] Américo JHP; Messias TG; Torres NH; Américo GHP. Desreguladores endócrinos no ambiente e seus efeitos na biota e saúde humana. Pesticidas: r. ecotoxicol. e meio ambiente, *Curitiba*, 2012, 22, 17-34.

[25] Lara, LAS; Duarte, AAF; Reis, RM. Impacto dos disruptores endócrinos na função reprodutiva e sexual de homens e mulheres. Rev.Bras. Ginecol Obstet., *Ribeirão Preto*, 2011, 33(12), 377-380.

[26] Svechnikov K; Stukenborg J; Savchuck I; Söder O. Similar causes of various reproductive disorders in early life. *Asian Journal of Andrololology*, 2014, 16: 50-69.

[27] Rittler, M; Castilla, EE. Endocrine disruptors and congenital anomalies. Cad. Saúde Pública, *Rio de Janeiro*, 2002, 18(2), 421-428.

[28] Fenton, SE; Reed, CE. Exposure to Diethylstilbestrol during Sensitive Life Stages: a legacy of heritable health effects. Birth Defects Res C Embryo Today, *Triangle Park Research*, 2013, 1-23.

[29] Sonnenschein, C; Soto, AM. Environmental causes of cancer: endocrine disruptors as carcinogens. *Nat Rev Endocrinol*, 2010, 6(7), 363-370.

[30] Patrick, L. Thyroid Disruption: Mechanisms and Clinical Implications in Human Health. *Alternative Medicine Review*, 2009, 14(4), 326-346.

[31] Murthy, BK; Murthy, MB. Thyroid disruptors and their possible clinical implications. *Indian J Pharmacol.*, 2012, 44(4), 542-543.

[32] Schneider, JE; Brozek, JM; Rhinehart, EK. Our stolen figures: The interface of sexual differentiation, endocrine disruptors, maternal programming, and energy balance. *Hormones and behavior*, 2014, 66, 104-119.

[33] Blumberg, B; Grun, F. Environmental Obesogens: Organotins and Endocrine Disruption via Nuclear Receptor Signaling. *Endocrinology*, 2006, 147(6), 50-55.

[34] Mayor RVG; Vidal AL; Caamano M; Giménez AL. Disruptores endocrinos y obesidad: obesógenos. *Endocrinol Nutr*, 2012, 59(4), 261-267.

[35] Gore, AC. Neuroendocrine targets of endocrine disruptors. *Hormones* (Athens), 2010, 9(1), 16-27.

[36] Carvalho CML; Campos AEST; Martins DS; Raposo AMF; Viveiros APR; Batoréu MCC. Dioxinas: origens e efeitos na população humana. Available from: http://www.ordembiologos/Biologias/N3.html. Biologias, 3, March, 2001. Accessed August, 2014.

In: Public Health and Harm Reduction
Editor: Meredith B. Morris
ISBN: 978-1-63482-159-9


*Chapter 4*

# TOBACCO PUBLIC HEALTH AND HARM REDUCTION: PRINCIPLES, PERCEPTIONS AND PROGRAMS

***Marcia Erazo[1]*, Maria Paz Bertoglia[1], Juan Guillermo Gormaz[2], Matías Libuy[1] and Carla Bertossi[1]***

[1]School of Public Health, Faculty of Medicine, University of Chile, Chile
[2]Molecular and Clinical Pharmacology Program, Institute of Biomedical Sciences, University of Chile, Chile

## ABSTRACT

Tobacco consumption is a worldwide epidemic that causes illness and mortality at all ages, sexes and countries. In order to protect population of damages of active and passive smoking, the World Health Organization (WHO), in accordance to the principles of the Charter of United Nations that promotes the right of people to enjoy the highest attainable standard of health without distinction of race, religion, and political belief, economic or social condition, developed a framework for tobacco control. The WHO Framework Convention on Tobacco Control (FCTC) is an international treaty that provides evidence-based recommendations for health promotion and tobacco control. Among the strategies that have been implemented worldwide to curve the epidemic of tobacco smoking are: smoking ban in public places, package labelling, to remove vending machines, health promotion for school-children and at workplaces, increase taxes, tobacco cessation programs, among others. Complete smoking ban in public places is a successful policy; several studies in different countries have shown a reduction in myocardial infarction after few months of the policy implementation. Other strategies have been less implemented and not fully evaluated. Limited political commitment and limited human capital expertise are examples of perceived barriers that were identified by countries to implement in a proper manner the FCTC. An increase in country capacity building and technical cooperation between countries are priorities to secure worldwide implementation of FCTC.

**Keywords:** Tobacco, public policies, smoking, health promotion

## Abbreviations

| | |
|---|---|
| ED | Emergency department |
| FCTC | Framework Convention on Tobacco Control |
| NoT | The Not-on-Tobacco program |
| NRT | Nicotine Replacement Therapy |
| STPs | School tobacco policies |
| SCH | Second Hand Smoking |
| TTMC | Transtheoretical Model of Change |
| WHO | World Health Organization |

## 1. Introduction

Tobacco consumption is a worldwide epidemic that causes illness and mortality at all ages, sexes and countries. Despite major successes in evidence-based tobacco control over the past 50 years, tobacco exposure remains one of the world's major health threats. In the 20th century, an estimated 100 million deaths were due to smoking [1] representing 16% of deaths among men and 7% of deaths among women [2]. It has been predicted that there will be one billion deaths attributable to tobacco in the 21st century [3] and it is likely that this burden will differentially affect women more than men due to women being at an earlier stage of the tobacco epidemic than men in most parts of the world [4] In order to protect population of damages of active and passive smoking, the World Health Organization (WHO), in accordance to the principles of the Charter of United Nations that promotes the right of people to enjoy the highest attainable standard of health without distinction of race, religion, and political belief, economic or social condition, developed a framework for tobacco control. The aim of this chapter is to show an updated version about the strategies on tobacco control and elucidate the main challenges to propose effective public policies against smoking.

## 2. STRATEGIES ON TOBACCO CONTROL

The WHO Framework Convention on Tobacco Control (FCTC) is an international treaty that provides evidence-based recommendations for health promotion and tobacco control. Among the strategies that have been implemented worldwide to curve the epidemic of tobacco smoking are: smoking ban in public places, package labelling, to remove vending machines, health promotion for school-children and at workplaces, increase taxes, tobacco cessation programs, among others. Complete smoking ban in public places is a successful policy because several studies in different countries have shown a reduction in myocardial infarction after few months of the policy implementation. Other strategies have been less implemented and not fully evaluated. In figure 1 is shown the main strategies on tobacco control.

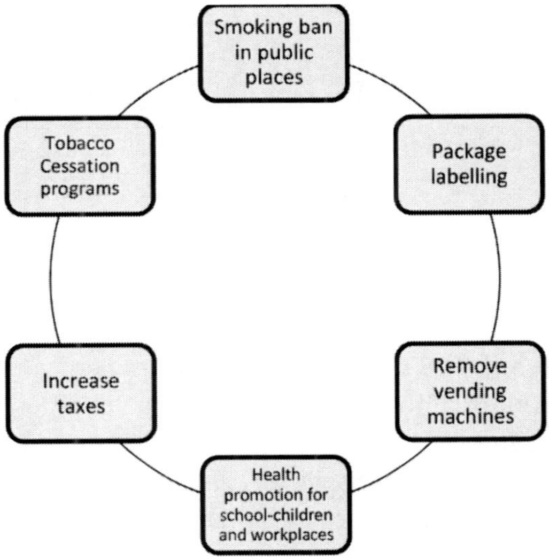


Figure 1. Strategies on tobacco control.

## 2.1. Smoking Ban in Public Places

WHO had categorized eight public places of interest for smoke-free legislation: healthcare facilities; educational facilities other than universities; universities; government facilities; indoor offices and workplaces; restaurants; pubs and bars; and public transport [5]. There is a wealth of research showing the health benefits to entire populations when communities implement comprehensive smokefree laws and/or regulations. These laws improve the health of hospitality workers and the general population by improving indoor air quality, reducing acute myocardial infarctions and asthma exacerbations, and improving infant and birth outcomes. Some studies report reduced smoking prevalence and cigarette consumption and improved cessation outcomes after smokefree legislation. In addition to the health benefits, economic studies confirm that smokefree laws do not adversely affect business revenues or operating costs. In Table 1 is shown evidence about the major benefits of smoking ban in public places [6].

**Table 1. Main benefits of smoking ban in public places**

| | [Reference] |
|---|---|
| Improve the health of hospitality workers and the general population by improving indoor air quality. | [7-20] |
| Reduce acute myocardial infarctions. | [20-23] |
| Reduce asthma exacerbations. | [24-26] |
| Improve infant birth outcomes. | [27,28] |
| Reduced smoking prevalence and cigarette consumption | [46-48] |
| Smokefree laws do not adversely affect business revenues or operating costs. | [29-38] |
| Improved cessation outcomes. | [39-45] |

A recent report about smokefree legislation in Scotland showed that comprehensive smoke-free legislation leads to an immediate and sustained reduction in exposure to secondhand smoke among workers in the hospitality sector, and both children and non-smoking adults in the general population [7]. In this line, a 32-country study of indoor air pollution revealed that countries with national smokefree indoor public places legislation had lower fine particle air pollution levels than those without restrictions [8]. Another air quality study in 128 Irish pubs in 15 countries revealed that fine particle air pollution was 93% lower in places where smoking was not permitted, compared to places that allowed smoking [9]. Declines in fine particle indoor air pollution ranging from 71% to 99% have been demonstrated after local, state, or national smokefree legislation in Lexington KY [10]; Boston [11]; Austin TX [12]; New York [13], Minneapolis [14], Massachusetts [15], Scotland [16] Ireland [17], England [18], Finland [19] and Italy [20].

### *Acute Myocardial Infarction*

Also is well known that smokefree enactments are associated with measurable reductions in heart attack rates and improvements in respiratory health. A meta-analysis of 17 studies in six countries found a pooled estimated reduction of 10% in the incidence of acute coronary events after the implementation of smoke-free legislation [20]. One systematic review and meta-analysis in the Journal of the American College of Cardiology reviewed 11 studies from ten locations worldwide and reported a 17% overall decline in AMIs after smokefree legislation, especially among younger and nonsmoking populations [21], with an incremental decline of 26% each year after implementation. Another meta-analysis of 12 studies/reports published in Circulation estimated that communities experience a 15% drop in heart attacks during the first year of smokefree legislation, with continued decline of 36% in 3 years [22]. Using simulation, one study predicts an immediate and significant 5%–15% reduction in AMI after smokefree legislation [23].

### *Asthma and Infant Birth Outcomes*

A mean reduction in the rate of hospitalizations for childhood asthma of 18% per year was observed in Scotland, following a comprehensive ban in 2006, compared with a mean annual rise of 5% before the ban [24]. In addition, Emergency department (ED) visits for asthma declined 22% from pre to post-law in Lexington, Kentucky, adjusting for seasonality, secular trends, and demographic characteristics [25]. There were fewer ED visits for asthma among both children and adults, with a more pronounced decline among adults (18% decline for those aged:19 years; 24% for those aged 20 years). Consistent with this population-based study, a convenience sample of 96 patients with asthma in Portugal reported positive improvements in asthma management (i.e., daily life activities, symptoms, and medication use) [26]. Of those who reported positive changes, nearly all were no longer exposed to SHS after the smokefree legislation. There also is emerging science on infant and birth outcomes and smokefree legislation. An analysis of the 1973–2003 Multiple Cause of Death Files from the National Center for Health Statistics reported a significant association between smokefree laws and Sudden Infant Death Syndrome (SIDS); smokefree restaurants and bar laws were associated with four fewer SIDS on average per year [27]. In regard to birth outcomes, there was a 25% decline in risk for preterm birth and a 12% decrease in maternal smoking 1 year after Ireland's law [28].

### *Businesses*

There is clear evidence that smokefree legislation does not hurt restaurant or bar businesses, and in some cases business may improve. There have been several published reviews of the economics of smokefree laws [2; 29]. Most of the economic impact studies have evaluated revenues and/or employment in the hospitality industry before and after smokefree legislation. Consistent with earlier economic impact studies, a Canadian study of retail sales tax data found no adverse effects on business after Ottawa's smokefree law went into effect in 2001[30]. Similarly, an analysis of California tax revenue data from 1990 – 2002 showed that restaurant and bar revenues increased, respectively, after the 1995 smokefree restaurant law and the 1998 smokefree bar law [31]. In this issue, Klein et al. [32] report no significant changes in bar or restaurant employment in rural and urban regions after Minnesota's statewide smokefree law business. Even in Lexington, Kentucky, located in a tobacco producing state with higher-than-average smoking levels, there was no economic harm after a 2004 smokefree law, [33] similar to other published studies [34,35]. No relationship was observed between the law and employment neither in contiguous counties nor between the smokefree law and business openings or closures in alcohol-serving and non–alcohol-serving businesses [33]. Three studies examined economic indicators other than revenues and employment. A study of one national restaurant chain's 23 Arizona restaurants showed that municipal smokefree laws did not have a significant effect on the probability of employee separation in the years after implementation [36]. It was expected that training costs associated with employee turnover would not rise for full-service restaurants in municipalities that enact smokefree laws. Similar findings were reported in South Australia [37]. Further, a study of sale prices of bars located in smokefree communities reported no difference in the sale price based on whether or not the community was smokefree [38].

### *Cessation Outcomes*

Seven studies reported positive effects of smokefree legislation on attempts to quit and/or cessation outcomes. Young U.S. adults living in states with smokefree private worksite laws were 4.6% more likely to quit smoking than those in states without these laws [39] laws are more likely to attempt to quit smoking and have more negative perceptions of smoking [40]. In

California, smokers in communities with comprehensive smokefree workplace ordinances were more likely to self-report that they quit within 6 months of the survey than those who live in communities with no smokefree laws [41]. In Ireland, 46% of smokers reported that the smokefree law had prompted them to attempt to quit [42]. Researchers studied the effect of Italy's smokefree law on efficacy of smoking cessation treatments. The smokefree law was associated with increased 12-month abstinence levels and motivation to quit, [43] and an 8% decrease in cigarette consumption within about 3 months post-law [44]. In New Zealand, monthly calls to the quitline77 and provision of NRT (Nicotine Replacement Therapy ) vouchers increased significantly in the 12 months after implementation of smokefree legislation, controlling for quitline advertising expenditures, print media coverage, and other smoking-related advertising expenditures [45].

***Prevalence***

It is widely known that voluntary, or private sector, smokefree policies reduce tobacco consumption and smoking prevalence [46], but far less is understood about the effects of smokefree laws on smoking prevalence in the general population. There is some evidence that declines in smoking may occur immediately after these laws go into effect, but these declines may not be sustained over time. Population-based studies and those with workers demonstrate that clean indoor air laws reduce adult smoking prevalence and/or cigarette consumption [47]. In an analysis of the Current Population Survey Tobacco Use Supplement, 1992–2002, strong state smokefree laws were estimated to decrease adult smoking prevalence by 11%, with greater effects for men/boys and those aged 25–39 years [48].

## 2.2. Increase Taxes

Tobacco excise taxes are known to be effective in reducing smoking at the population level [49,50]. These effects grow over time and lead to substantial savings in lives and health care costs [51]. Bowser et al., estimate the effect of tobacco taxes on total mortality and cause-specific mortality in the 50 States plus the District of Columbia, USA, over the period 1970-2005 as well as the net effect on deaths averted in 2010. The authors concluded that higher tobacco taxes lead to lower total mortality rates and avoided deaths. Strong tobacco tax policies are essential to improving overall population health [52]. A recent study showed that state cigarette taxes may be an effective population-level intervention to decrease racial/ethnic and socioeconomic disparities in maternal smoking during pregnancy. [53]. About the taxes as an effective intervention, Chaloupka FJ. et al., concluded that increases in cigarette taxes in countries with simpler tax structures will be more effective in reducing cigarette smoking and its health and economic consequences than comparable tax increases in countries where tax structures are more complicated and there are greater opportunities for switching to cheaper brands in order to avoid a tax increase [54].

## 2.3. Health Promotion for School-Children and Workplaces

A recent Cochrane's review showed that a study which compared two 'middle schools' from two different regions in China, with 1807 participants, did not significantly affect students' smoking behavior. The experimental conditions included the introduction of a tobacco policy, environmental changes, and communication activities, while the control condition was no intervention. After a year's follow-up the study found no differences in smoking prevalence between intervention and control schools. Also the authors concluded that the majority of 24 observational studies analyzed, reported that schools with highly enforced policies, smoking ban extended to outdoor spaces, involving teachers and including sanctions for transgressions, with assistance to quit for smokers plus support by prevention programs, did not show a significant difference in smoking prevalence, when compared to schools adopting weaker or no policies [55].

The workplace appears to be a useful setting for helping people to stop smoking. Large groups of smokers are available who can easily be reached and helped, using proven methods. It is also in the employers' interests to improve the health of their workforce. Recent changes introducing anti-smoking laws in many developed countries may have eased the pressure to demonstrate the value of work-based programs. The situation in developing countries still requires that such methods be tested and proved in those communities. In this line, Cahil K et al., in a recent Cochrane review, showed strong evidence that some interventions directed towards individual smokers increase the likelihood of quitting smoking. These include individual and group counselling, pharmacological treatment to overcome nicotine addiction, and multiple interventions targeting smoking cessation as the primary or only outcome. All these interventions show similar effects whether offered in the workplace or elsewhere. Self-help interventions and social support are less effective. Although people taking up these interventions are more likely to stop, the absolute numbers of individual who quit smoking are low [56].

## 2.4. Package Labelling

Health warnings on cigarette packages are among the most common means of communicating the health risks of smoking. However, few studies have evaluated the impact of package warnings on consumer knowledge about tobacco risks [57].

The extent to which smokers understand the magnitude of these health risks has a strong influence on their smoking behavior [58-60] Smokers who perceive greater health risk from smoking are more likely to intend to quit and to quit smoking successfully [61,62]. The health risks of smoking are also the most common motivation to quit cited by current and former smokers, as well as the best predictor of long-term abstinence among reasons for quitting [63-65].

Hammond et al., concluded significant gaps in the knowledge of the risks of smoking between participants from four developed countries. Smokers who noticed the warnings were significantly more likely to endorse health risks, including lung cancer and heart disease. However? Smokers are not fully informed about the risks of smoking. Warnings that are graphic, larger, and more comprehensive in content are more effective in communicating the health risks of smoking. [57]

On the other hand, longitudinal studies consistently suggest that exposure to tobacco advertising and promotion is associated with the likelihood that adolescents will start or no to smoke. Based on the strength and specificity of this association, evidence of a dose-response relationship, the consistency of findings across numerous observational studies, temporality of exposure and smoking behaviors observed, as well as the theoretical plausibility regarding the impact of advertising, we conclude that tobacco advertising and promotion increases the likelihood that adolescents will start or no to smoke [66].

## 2.5. Remove Vending Machines

Controlling access is an established strategy for reducing consumption of substances harmful to health, in particular tobacco, alcohol, and illicit drugs. Of adolescents who start smoking more than a third become daily smokers in secondary school [57]. Successful restriction of young people's access to tobacco products could help prevent them from developing this addiction [66]. Tobacco vending machines in public spaces (e.g., near schools, playgrounds, sports facilities) provided unhindered and anonymous access to cigarettes. It was not uncommon for children to purchase cigarettes from vending machines, despite the restriction on smoking [68]. Apart from its significance as a source of tobacco, the presence of vending machines within public spaces also normalized the perception of cigarettes and facilitated their acceptance. [69]. FCTC in their Article 16 advocates for two basic options concerning tobacco vending machines: limit access for adolescents or enact a total ban on tobacco vending machines. In this line, recent evidence concluded that electronic locking devices on cigarette vending machines alone are not effective and total ban on tobacco vending machines is the only suitable strategy to diminish tobacco consumption in young people. [69].

## 2.6. Tobacco Cessation Programs

Secker – Walker et al., concluded that although intervention communities often showed substantial awareness of their programs, this rarely led to higher quit smoking rates. Similarly, increased knowledge of health risks, changes in attitudes to smoking, more quitting attempts, and better environmental and social support for quitting were not accompanied by reductions in community smoking levels. In the best designed trials, light to moderate smokers did slightly better than heavy smokers (the US COMMIT study), and men did a little better than women (the Australian CART study), but overall smoking rates remained similar between intervention and control communities [70].

In this line, a recent Cochrane's review showed that interventions which are designed to help adolescent smokers to quit are generally effective. In particular the authors recommend programs that combine a variety of approaches, including taking into account the young person's preparation for quitting, supporting behavioral change and enhancing motivation show promise. Following Santon A et al., is possible to categorize the type of program by similar interventions, comparison groups and participants. This led to three main types of intervention, based on:

1) Transtheoretical Model of Change (TTMC): TTMC is a model of intentional change and focuses on the decision making of an individual.

2) Psychosocial interventions including motivational enhancement: Psychosocial interventions involve motivational interviewing, relapse prevention and resisting social and cultural pressures.
3) The Not-on-Tobacco program (NoT): The NoT program is a gender-specific group program implemented in schools or communities, drawing on social cognitive theory.

Pooled results from 3 TTMC studies demonstrated that there was a significant effect in favor of the intervention on smoking cessation (RR = 1.56, 95% CI 1.21 – 2.01). Pooled results from 12 Psychosocial interventions were also significantly in favor of the intervention (RR = 1.60. 95% CI 1.28 – 2.01). Pooled results from 6 NoT interventions demonstrated a marginally statistically significant effect of the intervention (RR = 1.31, 95% CI 1.01 to 1.71). However, none of the six NoT interventions demonstrated significant improvements individually.

Nevertheless, many of the studies were at a high risk of selection bias, in which groups or individuals were not randomly allocated. Secondly, several individual studies had low statistical power. In third place, many studies did not use gold standard techniques including biochemical measures of smoking cessation or sustained abstinence measures. These issues reduce the confidence in wider application of these results. To conclude, there is some evidence to suggest that complex interventions may be effective in increasing smoking cessation in young smokers. Future research should focus on direct comparisons between effective treatments [71].

## 3. Challenges on Tobacco Control

Limited political commitment and limited human capital expertise are examples of perceived barriers that were identified by countries to implement in a proper manner the FCTC. An increase in country capacity building and technical cooperation between countries are priorities to secure worldwide implementation of FCTC.

The Spanish case is an example that partial bans do not work, and that public health scientists and consumers can join forces to overcome social and limited political commitment. In 2006, legislation was enacted which prohibited smoking in enclosed public places, transportation and indoor workplaces. However, bars, cafes and restaurants were partially exempted. Smoking areas were allowed in premises with a floor space of over 100 $m^2$

and, if under 100 $m^2$, the proprietor could decide whether or not to allow smoking. This had the support of the tobacco industry and was promoted in a number of other countries as the 'Spanish model'. An evaluation of nicotine levels in the air and salivary concentrations of cotinine in hospitality workers before and after the ban in Spain showed that there were large reductions in levels in premises with strict bans. However, high levels remained where smoking was permitted, and in some cases, these were even higher than before the ban in designated smoking areas [72-73]. The continued risks to the health of hospitality workers were heavily publicized. Repeated public surveys showed over 70% support for a complete ban in bars and restaurants. As a result of intensive campaigning, the law was amended in 2010 and now smoking is prohibited in all enclosed bars and restaurants, healthcare services and educational centers (both indoors and outdoors), and outdoor children's playgrounds. Designated smoking rooms are permitted in mid- and long-stay psychiatric services, nursing homes, prisons and up to 30% of hotel rooms [74].

In Table 2 is shown a priority future research which must include the effects of smokefree laws. This research evidence is critically important for health advocates, responsible for translating and disseminating science to policymakers. Funding agencies need to target these research priorities in order to provide a science base for smokefree legislation that protects [6].

**Table 2. Priority future research: effects of smokefree laws**

| |
|---|
| (1) Population and worker health indicators such as asthma and COPD |
| (2) Outdoor tobacco smoke exposure |
| (3) Air pollution, considering strength of and time since smokefree legislation |
| (4) Smoking prevalence and smoking cessation, especially in vulnerable populations including racial/ethnic minorities and those living in rural communities, considering strength of and time since law |
| (5) Cross-border economic effects of smokefree laws, considering community-level socioeconomic variation |
| (6) Low-income populations, women, racial/ethnic minorities, and older adults. |
| (7) Smoking at the home, considering non-smokers who live with smokers, including many children, continued to be exposed to high levels of second-hand smoke. |

## Conclusion

There is clear evidence that smokefree legislation does not hurt restaurant or bar businesses, did not have a significant effect on the probability of employee and in some cases business may improve. In this line, tobacco excise taxes are known to be effective in reducing smoking prevalence at the population level. These effects grow over time and lead to substantial savings in lives and health care costs. Smoke-free legislation can be remarkably effective; nevertheless the political and social obstacles to introducing and implementing effective smoke-free legislation can be considerable.

The tobacco industry presence and control in the retail environment is significant. Tobacco companies overwhelmingly provided tobacco gantries in the shops surveyed and influenced displays through a combination of requirements and incentives. The extensive involvement of tobacco companies in providing and monitoring retail displays suggests the importance of implementing policies to end this form of advertising.

## References

[1] Peto R, Lopez AD, Boreham J, Thun M, Heath C Jr. Mortality from tobacco in developed countries: indirect estimation from national vital statistics. *Lancet* 1992;339:1268–1278.

[2] Eriksen M, Chaloupka F. The economic impact of clean indoor air laws. *Cancer J Clinicians* 2007;57:367–78.

[3] WHO Report on the Global Tobacco Epidemic, 2008: the MPOWER package. Geneva: *World Health Organization,* 2008.

[4] Lopez AD, Collishaw NE, Piha T. A descriptive model of the cigarette epidemic in developed countries. *Tob Control* 1994;3:242–247.

[5] WHO. Framework Convention on Tobacco Control. World Health Organisation, http://www.who.int/tobacco/framework/WHO_FCTC_english.pdf; 2003. p. 8.

[6] Hahn E, Lee K, Okoli C, Troutman A, Powell R. Smoke-free laws and indoor air pollution in Lexington and Louisville. *Louisville Med* 2005; 52:391– 394, 409, 415.

[7] NHS Health Scotland. Evaluation of the Scottish Smoke-free legislation http://www.healthscotland.com/scotlands-health/evidence/Smokefree legislation.aspx.

[8] Hyland A, Travers MJ, Dresler C, Higbee C, Cummings KM. A 32-country comparison of tobacco smoke derived particle levels in indoor public places. *Tob Control* 2008;17:159–165.

[9] Connolly GN, Carpenter CM, Travers MJ, Cummings KM, Hyland A, Mulcahy M, Clancy L. How smoke-free laws improve air quality: a global study of Irish pubs. *Nicotine Tob Res* 2009;11:600 –605.

[10] Repace JL, Hyde JN, Brugge D. Air pollution in Boston bars before and after a smoking ban. *BMC Public Health* 2006;6:266.

[11] Waring MS, Siegel JA. An evaluation of the indoor air quality in bars before and after a smoking ban in Austin, Texas. *J Expo Sci Environ Epidemiol* 2007;17:260–268.

[12] CDC. Indoor air quality in hospitality venues before and after implementation of a clean indoor air law—Western New York, 2003.

[13] Bohac DL, Hewett MJ, Kapphahn, KI, Grimsrud DT, Apte MG, Gundel LA. Change in indoor particle levels after a smoking ban in Minnesota bars and restaurants. *Am J Prev Med* 2010; 39:S3–S9.

[14] Alpert HR, Carpenter CM, Travers MJ, Connolly GN. Environmental and economic evaluation of the Massachusetts Smoke-Free Workplace Law. *J Community Health* 2007;32:269–281.

[15] Semple S, Creely KS, Naji A, Miller BG, Aynes JG. Secondhand smoke levels in Scottish pubs: the effect of smoke-free legislation. *Tob Control* 2007;16:127–132.

[16] Goodman P, Agnew M, McCaffrey M, Paul G, Clancy L. Effects of the Irish smoking ban on respiratory health of bar workers and air quality in Dublin pubs. *Am J Resp Crit Care Med* 2007;175:840 –845.

[17] Gotz NK, van Tongeren M, Wareing H, Wallace LM, Semple S, Maccalman L. Changes in air quality and second-hand smoke exposure in hospitality sector businesses after introduction of the English Smoke-free legislation. *J Public Health* (Oxf) 2008;30:421– 428.

[18] Johnsson T, Tuomi T, Riuttala H, Hyvärinen M, Rothberg M, Reijula K. Environmental tobacco smoke in Finnish restaurants and bars before and after smoking restrictions were introduced. *Ann Occup Hyg* 2006;50:331– 341.

[19] Valente P, Forastiere F, Bacosi A, Cattani G, Di Carlo S, Ferri M, Figà-Talamanca I, Marconi A, Paoletti L, Perucci C, Zuccaro P. Exposure to fine and ultrafine particles from secondhand smoke in public places before and after the smoking ban, Italy 2005. *Tob Control* 2007;16:312–317.

[20] Mackay DF, Irfan MO, Haw S, Pell JP. Meta-analysis of the effect of comprehensive smoke-free legislation on acute coronary events. *Heart.* 2010;96:1525-1530.

[21] Meyers DG, Neuberger JS, He J. Cardiovascular effect of bans on smoking in public places: a systematic review and meta-analysis. *Jam Coll Cardiol* 2009;54:1249 –1255.

[22] Lightwood JM, Glantz SA. Declines in acute myocardial infarction after smoke-free laws and individual risk attributable to secondhand smoke. *Circulation* 2009;120:1373–1379.

[23] Richiardi L, Vizzini L, Merletti F, Barone-Adesi F. Cardiovascular benefits of smoking regulations: the effect of decreased exposure to passive smoking. *Prev Med* 2009;48:167–172.

[24] Mackay DF, Haw S, Ayres JG, Pell JP. Smoke-free legislation and hospitalizations for childhood asthma. *N Engl J Med* 2010;363:1139e45.

[25] Rayens MK, Burkhart PV, Zhang M, Lee S, Moser DK, Mannino D, Hahn EJ. Reduction in asthma related emergency department visits after implementation of a smoke-free law. *J Allergy Clin Immunol* 2008;122:537– 541.e3.

[26] Areias A, Duarte J, Figueiredo J, Lucas R, Matos I, Pires J, Fonseca AG, Castanheira JL. Asthma and the new antismoking legislation. What has changed? *Rev Port Pneumol* 2009;15:27– 42.

[27] Markowitz S. The effectiveness of cigarette regulations in reducing cases of Sudden Infant Death Syndrome. *J Health Econ* 2008; 27:106 – 133.

[28] Kabir Z, Clarke V, Conroy R, McNamee E, Daly S, Clancy L. Low birthweight and preterm birth rates 1 year before and after the Irish workplace smoking ban. *BJOG* 2009;116:1782–1787.

[29] Scollo M, Lal A, Hyland A, Glantz S. Review of the quality of studies on the economic effects of smoke-free policies on the hospitality industry. *Tob Control* 2003;12:13–20.

[30] Luk R, Ferrence R, Gmel G. The economic impact of a smoke-free bylaw on restaurant and bar sales in Ottawa, Canada. *Addiction* 2006;101:738–745.

[31] Cowling DW, Bond P. Smoke-free laws and bar revenues in California—the last call. *Health Econ* 2005;14:1273– 1281.

[32] Klein EG, Forster JL, Collins N, Erickson DJ, Toomey TL. Employment change for bars and restaurants following a statewide clean indoor air policy. *Am J Prev Med* 2010;39:S16 –S22.

[33] Pyles MK, Mullineaux DJ, Okoi CTC, Hahn EJ. Economic impact of a smoke-free law in a tobacco-growing community. *Tob Control* 2007;16:66–68.

[34] CDC. Impact of a smoking ban on restaurant and bar revenues—El Paso, Texas, 2002. *MMWR Morb Mortal Wkly Rep* 2004;53: 150 –152.

[35] Scollo M, Lal A. Summary of studies assessig the economic impact of smoke-free policies in the hospitality industry. Melbourne, Australia: *VicHealth Centre for Tobacco Control*, 2008.

[36] Thompson E, Hahn E, Blomquist G, Garen J, Mullineaux D, Ogunro N, Rayens A. Smoke-free laws and employee turnover. *Contemp Econ Policy* 2008;26:351–359.

[37] Wakefield M, Siahpush M, Scollo M, Lal A, Hyland A, McCaul K, Miller C. The effect of a smoke-free law on restaurant business in South Australia. *Aust N Z J Public Health* 2002;26:375– 382.

[38] Alamar B, Glantz SA. Effect of smoke-free laws on bar value and profits. *Am J Public Health* 2007;97:1400 –1402.

[39] Tauras JA. Public policy and smoking cessation among young adults in the U.S. Health Policy 2004;68:321–332.

[40] Albers AB, Siegel M, Cheng DM, Biener L, Rigotti NA. Effect of smoking regulations in local restaurants on smokers' anti-smoking attitudes and quitting behaviours. *Tob Control* 2007;16:101– 106.

[41] Moskowitz JM, Lin Z, Hudes ES. The impact of workplace smoking ordinances in California on smoking cessation. *Am J Public Health* 2000;90:757– 761.

[42] Fong GT, Hyland A, Borland R, Hammond D, Hastings G, McNeill A, Anderson S, Cummings KM, Allwright S, Mulcahy M, Howell F, Clancy L, Thompson ME, Connolly G, Driezen P. Reductions in tobacco smoke pollution and increases in support for smoke-free public places following the implementation of comprehensive smoke-free workplace legislation in the Republic of Ireland: findings from the ITC Ireland/ UK survey. *Tob Control* 2006;15:iii51–iii58.

[43] Grassi MC, Enea D, Ferketich AK, Lu B, Nencini P. A smoking ban in public places increases the efficacy of bupropion and counseling o cessation outcomes at 1 year. *Nicotine Tob Res* 2009;11:1114 –1121.

[44] Gallus S, Zuccaro P, Colombo P, Apolone G, Pacifici R, Garattini S, La Vecchia C. Effects of new smoking regulations in Italy. *Ann Oncology* 2006;17:346 –347.

[45] Wilson N, Sertsou G, Edwards R, Thomson G, Grigg M, Li J. A new national smokefree law increased calls to a national quitline. *BMC Public Health* 2007;7:75.

[46] Hopkins DP, Razi S, Leeks KD, Priya Kalra G, Chattopadhyay SK, Soler RE; Task Force on Community Preventive Services. Smokefree policies to reduce tobacco use a systematic review. *Am J Prev Med* 2010;38:S275–S289.

[47] Dinno A, Glantz S. Tobacco control policies are egalitarian: a vulnerabilities perspective on clean indoor air laws, cigarette prices, and tobacco use disparities. *Soc Sci Med* 2009;68:1439–1447.

[48] Gerlowski DA, Levy DT, Tauras JA, Compton, C. The decision to smoke and the frequency of smoking by age and gender. *J Applied Econ Pol* 2009;28:1–19.

[49] Ross H1, Stoklosa M, Krasovsky K. Economic and public health impact of 2007-2010 tobacco tax increases in Ukraine. *Tob Control.* 2012;21:429-435.

[50] Kostova D, Andes L, Erguder T, Yurekli A, Keskinkılıç B, Polat S, Culha G, Kilinç EA, Taştı E, Erşahin Y, Ozmen M, San R, Ozcebe H, Bilir N, Asma S; Office on Smoking and Health, National Center for Chronic Disease Prevention and Health Promotion, CDC. Cigarette prices and smoking prevalence after a tobacco tax increase--Turkey, 2008 and 2012. *MMWR Morb Mortal Wkly Rep*. 2014 May 30;63:457-456.

[51] Levy DT1, Wen CP, Chen TY, Oblak M. Increasing taxes to reduce smoking prevalence and smoking attributable mortality in Taiwan: results from a tobacco policy simulation model. *Tob Control.* 2005;14 Suppl 1:i45-50.

[52] Bowser D1, Canning D2, Okunogbe A3. The impact of tobacco taxes on mortality in the USA, 1970-2005. *Tob Control.* 2014 Oct 28. pii: tobaccocontrol-2014-051666.

[53] Hawkins SS1, Baum CF. Impact of state cigarette taxes on disparities in maternal smoking during pregnancy. *Am J Public Health.* 2014;104:1464-1470.

[54] Chaloupka FJ1, Kostova D, Shang C. Cigarette excise tax structure and cigarette prices: evidence from the global adult tobacco survey and the U.S. National Adult Tobacco Survey. *Nicotine Tob Res*. 2014;16 Suppl 1:S3-9

[55] Coppo A, Galanti M, Giordano L, Buscemi D, Bremberg S, Faggiano F. School policies for preventing smoking among young people. *Cochrane Database of Systematic Reviews* 2014, Issue 10.

[56] Cahill K, Lancaster T. Workplace interventions for smoking cessation. Cochrane Database of Systematic Reviews 2014, Issue 2. Art. No.: CD003440.

[57] Hammond D, Fong GT, McNeill A, Borland R, Cummings KM. Effectiveness of cigarette warning labels in informing smokers about the risks of smoking: findings from the International Tobacco Control (ITC) Four Country Survey *Tob Control* 2006;15:iii19-iii25

[58] Janz N, Becker MH. The health belief model: a decade later. *Health Educ Q* 1984;11:1–47.

[59] Bandura A. Self-efficacy: toward a unifying theory of behavioral change. *Psychol Rev* 1977;84:191–215.

[60] Ajzen I. The theory of planned behavior. *Organ Behav Hum Decis Process* 1991;50:179–211.

[61] Nourjah P, Wagener DK, Eberhardt M, Horowitz AM. Knowledge of risk factors and risk behaviours related to coronary heart disease among blue and white collar males. *J Public Health Policy* 1994;15:443–459.

[62] Romer D, Jamieson P. The role of perceived risk in starting and stopping smoking. In: Slovic, ed. Smoking: risk, perception, and policy. *Thousand Oaks California: Sage,* 2001;65–80.

[63] Curry SJ, Grothaus L, McBride C. Reasons for quitting: intrinsic and extrinsic motivation for smoking cessation in a population-based sample of smokers. *Addict Behav* 1997;22:727–739.

[64] Hammond D, McDonald PW, Fong GT, Brown KS, Cameron R. The impact of cigarette warning labels and smoke-free bylaws on smoking cessation: evidence from former smokers. *Can J Public Health* 2004;95:201–4.

[65] Hyland A, Li Q, Bauer JE, Giovino GA, Steger C, Cummings KM. Predictors of cessation in a cohort of current and former smokers followed over 13 years. *Nicotine Tob Res* 2004;6(suppl 3):S363–69.

[66] Lovato C, Watts A, Stead LF. Impact of tobacco advertising and promotion on increasing adolescent smoking behaviours. *Cochrane Database of Systematic Reviews 2011, Issue 10.* Art. No.: CD003439.

[67] US Centers for Disease Control and Prevention. Selected cigarette smoking initiation and quitting behaviors among high school students—United States, 1997. *MMWR Morbid Mortal Wkly Rep* 1998;47:386–389.

[68] German Cancer Research Center. Tabaksteuererhöhungen - fakten und argumente. *Heidelberg, Germany: German Cancer Research Center,* 2003: 1–3.

[69] Schneider S, Meyer C, Yamamoto S, Solle D. Implementation of electronic locking devices for adolescents at German tobacco vending machines: intended and unintended changes of supply and demand. *Tob Control.* 2009;18:294-301

[70] Secker-Walker R, Gnich W, Platt S, Lancaster T. Community interventions for reducing smoking among adults. *Cochrane Database of Systematic Reviews 2002, Issue 3.* Art. No.: CD001745.

[71] Stanton A, Grimshaw G.Tobacco cessation interventions for young people. *Cochrane Database Syst Rev.* 2013;8:CD003289

[72] Nebot N, López MJ, Ariza C, Pérez-Ríos M, Fu M, Schiaffino A, Muñoz G, Saltó E, Fernández E. Impact of the Spanish smoking law on exposure to secondhand smoke in offices and hospitality venues: before and after study. *Environ Health Perspect* 2009;117:344e7.

[73] Fernández E, Fu M, Pascual JA, López MJ, Pérez-Ríos M, Schiaffino A, Martínez-Sánchez JM, Ariza C, Saltó E, Nebot M. Impact of the Spanish smoking control law on exposure to second-hand smoke and respiratory health in hospitality workers: a cohort study. *Plos ONE* 2009;4:e4244.

[74] Gruer L, Tursan d'Espaignet E, Haw S, Fernández E, Mackay J. Smoke-free legislation: global reach, impact and remaining challenges. *Public Health.* 2012;126:227-229.

In: Public Health and Harm Reduction
Editor: Meredith B. Morris

ISBN: 978-1-63482-159-9


*Chapter 5*

# SMOKING-RELATED DISENGAGEMENT BELIEFS AMONG SMOKING ASTHMA PATIENTS

***Efrat Neter*[*], *Gal Gida and Ella Eliya***
Ruppin Academic Center, Israel

## ABSTRACT

*Background:* Though smoking accelerates asthma, smoking is actually more common among asthmatics. A possible explanation for this discrepancy is that asthmatics use more techniques such as disengagement beliefs to reduce the dissonance between their knowledge on the deleterious effects of smoking and their behavior. Disengagement beliefs are beliefs that minimize the behavior and are generated in order to explain / justify non-congruent behaviors

*Methods:* Participants (n= 199, 94 asmathics and 105 non-asthmatics filled out a self-reported on-line questionnaire measuring disengagement beliefs (Dijkstra, 2009; 12 items, α = .84) and the Brief Illness Perception Questionnaire (IPQ-B, Broadbent, Petrie, Main, & Weinman, 2006). Disengagement beliefs were predicted by two independent variables: Asthma and smoking status.

*Results:* Smokers (M=3.39) used significantly more smoking-related disengagement beliefs than non smokers (M=2.55). An interaction between smoking and asthma status was significant so that asthmatic

[*] Corresponding author: neter@ruppin.ac.il.

smokers (M=3.66) held significantly more smoking-related disengagement beliefs than non-asthmatic smokers (M=3.12) and all other combinations. Additionally, asthmatic smokers reported significantly less control over their illness and a significantly poorer understanding of their disease than non-smoking asthmatics. In contrast to the hypothesis, asthmatic smokers reported experiencing more symptoms and more consequences to their illness than non-smoking asthmatics.

*Conclusion:* Increased use of smoking-related disengagement beliefs among asthmatic smokers has limited impact, as indicated in the higher level of perceived consequences and reported symptoms of the illness among them, compared to non-smoking asthmatics. Disengagement beliefs provide an explanation for the seeming contradiction between smoking and asthma, and may provide clues for future interventions.

Though the detrimental effects of smoking are well-known, smoking is more prevalent among individuals with asthma than those without (Eisner, 2001; Mcleish & Zvolensky, 2010; Thomson, Chaudhuri, & Livingston 2004), and this holds also among adolescents (Precht, Keiding, & Madsen, 2012). In a review on smoking and asthma, Mcleish & Zvolensky (2010) report that smoking is a risk candidate for the development of asthma. Moreover, numerous studies found that among adults with persistent asthma active smoking is associated with more asthma symptoms, decreased asthma control, increased hospitalizations and ultimately increased risk of mortality (Eiser & Iribarren, 2006; Mcleish & Zvolensky, 2010; Shavit, Swern, Dong, Newcomb, Sazonov Kocevar, & Taylor, 2007; Silverman, Boudreaux, Woodruff, Clark, & Camargo, 2012; Siroux, Pin, Oryszczyn, Le Moual, & Kauffmann, 2000; Thomson, Chaudhuri, & Livingston 2004). Evidence indicates that cigarette smoking has a persistent and dose-dependent, negative impact on the response to treatment (Niedoszytko, Gruchala-niedoszytko, Chelminska, Sieminska, Jassem, 2008). Conversely, smoking cessation is associated with improvements in lung functioning and asthma symptoms (To, Daly, Feldman, & McLimont, 2012). To summarize, asthma and active cigarette smoking interact to cause more severe symptoms, accelerated decline in lung function and impaired short-term therapeutic response to corticosteroids (Thomson, Chaudhuri, & Livingston, 2004).

People with asthma, possibly more than ordinary smokers, experience a conflict between their desire/need to smoke and their knowledge about the detrimental effects of smoking. The increased conflict is probably due to the experience of asthma. This inconsistency between their cognitions (e.g., adverse effects of smoking, long term goal of health) and their behavior results in a negative aroused state of cognitive dissonance (Festinger, 1957). In order to lessen this dissonance, people activate exempting/disengaging beliefs about smoking (Bandura, 1986; Chapman, Wong & Smith, 1993; Oakes, Chapman, Borland, Balmford, & Trotter 2004). An example to such thoughts is: "You have to die from something". Dijkastra (2009) notes that such cognitions lower the perception of the health risk, thereby providing peace of mind and preserving the indulgent behavior. This strategy of disengagement beliefs may provide an insight into the seeming contradiction between smoking and asthma.

Previous research on disengagement beliefs and smoking found that fewer smokers, compared to non-smokers, accept that smoking causes disease, and that smokers harbor self-exempting beliefs (e.g., "many people who smoke all their lives live to ripe age, so smoking is not all that bad for you") (Chapman, Wong & Smith, 1993). Dijkastra (2009) found that smokers with strong disengagement beliefs who experienced negative affect upon encountering persuasive messages against smoking were less likely to quit smoking.

The present work focused on smoking-related disengagements beliefs among smokers, and smoking asthma patients in particular. Prevalence of disengagement beliefs was first examined, hypothesizing that smokers will hold more disengagement beliefs than non-smokers and that asthma patients will hold more of these beliefs than non-asthmatics. An interaction between smoking and asthma status was hypothesized so that smoking asthmatics will hold the highest level of smoking-related disengagement beliefs. Past smokers were hypothesized to hold the middle ground between smokers and non-smokers. The present work went beyond disengagement beliefs to how people perceive their condition. Specifically, it was hypothesized that the disengagement beliefs will color the perceptions of asthma among asthma patients. Illness perceptions describe how patients view their illness (Petrie & Weinman, 1997), focusing on identity – the label and symptoms experienced as part of the illness; cause – the causal attributions patients make for their illness (physiological, genetic, psychological); timeline – whether the illness is chronic, acute or cyclical in nature; consequences – the beliefs in the seriousness of the illness; cure/control – beliefs about recovery from or controllability of the illness/symptoms and understanding of the disease. The present work focused on four main perceptions: consequences, identity (=symptoms), control, and understanding.

It was hypothesized that smoking asthmatics, in an attempt to minimize the contradiction between their smoking and its effect, will minimize the consequences and symptoms of the disease. Likewise, it was hypothesized that they will perceived their control and understanding to be lower than would former smokers and never smokers.

# METHODS

## Participants and Procedure

The study included 199 adults, 121 women and 78 men, ranging 20-50 in age (M=26.4). Ninety-four were individuals with asthma (44 of them smoking, 33 never-smokers, and 17 former smokers), and 105 were non-asthmatics (43 smokers, 38 never-smokers, and 24 former smokers). Participants were recruited through Internet forums and social networks, and a link to an on-line questionnaire was mailed to them.

# MATERIALS

**Smoking and asthma status.** One item tapped whether participants currently smoke/smoked in the past/never smoked, and another item tapped whether participants have asthma or not.

**Disengagement beliefs.** A 12-items questionnaire (Dijkstra, 2009) tapping reasons/rationalizations why it could be acceptable to smoke was used. Examples of items are: “I know heavy smokers who lived long” and “I have to die of something”. Ratings were made on a 5-point scale ranging from 'I do not agree' (1) to 'I agree' (5). Cronbach's alpha for the composite measure was = 0.84.

**Perception of Asthma**. Brief IPQ (Broadbent, Petrie, Main, &Weinman, 2006), a nine-item scale designed to rapidly assess the cognitive and emotional representations of illness, was used to assess the perception of asthma only among asthmatics.

# DATA ANALYSIS

Descriptive statistics on compensatory health beliefs were computed by smoking and asthma status and then tested for differences between groups.

Illness perception of asthma was compared between the smoking groups only among asthmatic patients.

# RESULTS

## Disengagement Beliefs by Smoking Status and Asthma Status

Table 1 displays the means (and SD) of disengagement beliefs by smoking and asthma status. As can be seen, the highest degree of disengagement beliefs is held among smokers, the least among never smokers, and past smokers are in between. People with asthma who smoke hold the highest degree of disengagement beliefs, whereas people with asthma who never smoked or who smoked in the past hold the lowest levels of disengagement beliefs. People with no asthma hold intermediate levels of disengagement beliefs; among them, never smokers hold these beliefs the least. A two-way ANOVA on disengagement beliefs by smoking and asthma status yielded a significant smoking effect, $F(2,196) = 30.00$, $p = .000$ ($\eta^2 = .24$), a significant asthma effect $F(1,197) = 10.99$, $p = .001$ ($\eta^2 = .05$), and a significant interaction $F(2,193) = 21.39$, $p = .001$ ($\eta^2 = .18$).

## Illness Perception among Asthma Patients by Smoking Status

Perceptions of asthma are displayed in Table 2. The perceptions include consequences, control, symptoms and understanding, hypothesized to be lower among smokers, as compared to the former smokers and never smokers. The results indicate that perceived control over the illness and understanding asthma were, as hypothesized, significantly lower among the smokers than past smokers and never smokers groups, $F(2,91) = 14.04$, $p = .000$ for control and $F(2,91) = 12.74$, $p = .028$, for understanding the illness. A planned contrast comparing the smoking group to the other two groups also yielded a significant difference, $t(91)=5.00$, $p=.000$ for control and $t(91)=2.69$, $p=.009$ for understanding asthma.

However, even though the smoking groups were significantly different on perceptions of consequences and symptoms ($F(2,91) = 5.27$, $p = .007$ for consequences and $F(2,91) = 3.53$, $p = .033$, for symptoms), the direction of the differences was such that smokers and past smokers perceived the consequences of asthma as more severe than never smokers, and smokers perceived the symptoms as more severe than both past smokers and never smokers.

# DISCUSSION

The purpose of the study was to examine the use of smoking-related disengagement beliefs among smoking asthmatics by comparing them to other groups related to smoking and asthma status, and this is the first study to do so.

The first hypothesis posited that smokers will employ more disengagement beliefs than non-smokers. The hypothesis was confirmed, and the finding is in line with previous studies which documented that smokers use different kinds of perceptions to justify their continued smoking (Chapman, Wong, & Smith, 1993; Dijkstra, 2009; Johnson, 1968; Oakes et al., 2004; Wakefield et al., 2008). The process starts with smokers being cognizant of smoking as harmful to their health; this realization creates an incompatibility between their beliefs and behavior, instigating a cognitive dissonance (Festinger, 1957). In order to decrease the cognitive dissonance, smokers then use the technique of disengagement beliefs which justifies their consumption of cigarettes.

**Table 1. Disengagement beliefs (M, SD) by smoking and asthma status**

| Smoking status | Asthmatic | Non-asthmatic | Overall |
|---|---|---|---|
| Smoker | 3.66 (.67) | 3.12 (.58) | 3.39 (.68) |
| Past smoker | 2.27 (1.00) | 3.31 (.49) | 2.78 (.90) |
| Never smoked | 2.29 (.63) | 2.82 (.82) | 2.55 (.78) |

**Table 2. Illness perception among asthma patients by smoking status (scale: 1-10)**

| Perceptions | Smokers | Past smokers | Never smokers |
|---|---|---|---|
| Consequences | 6.25 (2.19) | 6.29 (1.80) | 4.94 (1.44) |
| Control | 5.86 (2.02) | 7.88 (1.93) | 8.24 (2.21) |
| Symptoms | 6.32 (2.09) | 5.94 (1.56) | 5.24 (1.32) |
| Understanding | 7.32 (1.85) | 8.41 (2.15) | 8.33 (1.67) |

The second hypothesis posited that within the smoking group, people with asthma – the ones who feel the consequences of smoking the most - will harbor higher disengagement beliefs than non-asthmatic individuals. This hypothesis on the interaction between smoking and asthma status was also confirmed. It is possible that the severe health consequences of smoking make these smokers feel a cognitive dissonance at a higher level, hence the need for more disengagement beliefs (Van Zundert et al., 2008).

The illness perceptions related to asthma indicate that the use of disengagement beliefs has limited effect. Indeed, as hypothesized, smoking asthmatics understand their illness less than non or past smokers and also feel they have less control over it, another manifestation of compensatory belief. However, the present findings indicate, contrary to what was initially hypothesized, that smoking asthmatics feel more symptoms of asthma and also harsher consequences of asthma than the other two groups. These findings can be attributed to previous research indicating that smoking undermines the effectiveness of asthma medication and exacerbate asthmatic symptoms (Chalmers et al., 2002; Chaudhuri, Livingston, McMahon, Thomson, Borland, & Thomson, 2003).

It is noteworthy that smoking asthmatics understand their disease to a lesser extent than non-smokers and past smokers. This is an opening for persuasive communication related to the harmful effects of smoking, even specifically targeting disengagement beliefs. Indeed, Dijkstra (2009) found that smokers who strongly adhered to disengagement beliefs showed significantly more quitting activity when they received a persuasive message compared to smokers who adhered less to disengagement beliefs. Apparently, the disengagement beliefs do not harbor sufficient validity to withstand sound persuasive messages on the health consequences of smoking.

The findings of the current study are limited by its methods. Specifically, the sample of participants is a convenience sample, possibly biasing the kind of people who agreed to participate in the study. Second, the study used self reports; though these can hardly be avoided when beliefs and perception are the object of study, self reports may be augmented by other measurement methods.

In summary, the study focused on disengagement beliefs among smokers, documenting the paradox that smoking asthmatics hold the highest level of such beliefs. This finding calls for action, focusing and targeting these beliefs when treating smoking asthmatics.

## References

Bandura, A. (1986). *Social foundations of thought and action: A social cognitive theory*. Prentice-Hall, Inc.

Chalmers, G., Macleod, K., Little, S., Thomson, L., McSharry, C. & Thomson, N. (2002). Influence of cigarette smoking on inhaled corticosteroid treatment in mild asthma. *Thorax*, *57*(3), 226-230.

Chapman, S., Wong, W. L. & Smith, W. (1993). Self-exempting beliefs about smoking and health: differences between smokers and ex-smokers. *American Journal of Public Health*, *83*(2), 215-219.

Dijkstra, A. (2009). Disengagement beliefs in smokers: Do they influence the effects of a tailored persuasive message advocating smoking cessation? *Psychology & Health*, *24*(7), 791-804. doi: 10.1080/08870440801998962

Eisner, M. D., Yelin, E. H., Trupin, L. & Blanc, P. D. (2001). Asthma and smoking status in a population-based study of California adults. *Public Health Reports*, *116*(2), 148.

Eisner, M. D. & Iribarren, C. (2007). The influence of cigarette smoking on adult asthma outcomes. *Nicotine Tob Research*, *9*, 53–56.

Festinger, L. (1957). A theory of cognitive dissonance. Stanford University Press.

McLeish, A. C. & Zvolensky, M. J. (2010). Asthma and cigarette smoking: A review of the empirical literature. *Journal of Asthma*, *47*(4), 345-361.

Niedoszytko, M., Gruchala-Niedoszytko, M., Chelminska, M., Sieminska, A. & Jassem, E. (2008). Persistent impact of cigarette smoking on asthma. *Journal of Asthma*, *45*(6), 495-499.

Oakes, W., Chapman, S., Borland, R., Balmford, J. & Trotter, L. (2004). "Bulletproof skeptics in life's jungle": Which self-exempting beliefs about smoking most predict lack of progression towards quitting? *Preventive Medicine*, *39*(4), 776-782.

Petrie, K. J. & Weinman, J. (1997). Perceptions of health and illness: Current research and applications. Amsterdam: Harwood Academic Publishers.

Precht, D. H., Keiding, L. & Madsen, M. (2003). Smoking patterns among adolescents with asthma attending upper secondary schools: A community-based study. *Pediatrics*, *111*(5), 562.

Silverman, R. A., Boudreaux, E. D., Woodruff, P. G., Clark, S. & Camargo, C. A. (2003). Cigarette smoking among asthmatic adults presenting to 64 emergency departments. *CHEST Journal*, *123*(5), 1472-1479.

Siroux, V., Pin, I., Oryszczyn, M., Le Moual, N. & Kauffmann, F. (2000). Relationships of active smoking to asthma and asthma severity in the

EGEA study; Epidemiological study on the genetics and environment of asthma. *European Respiratory Journal*, *15*(3), 470-477.

Thomson, N. C., Chaudhuri, R. & Livingston, E. (2004). Asthma and cigarette smoking. *European Respiratory Journal*, *24*, 822–833.

To, T., Daly, C., Feldman, R. & McLimont, S. (2012). Results from a community-based program evaluating the effect of changing smoking status on asthma symptom control. *BMC public health*, *12*(1), 293.

In: Public Health and Harm Reduction
Editor: Meredith B. Morris
ISBN: 978-1-63482-159-9


*Chapter 6*

# PUBLIC HEALTH AND WASTE MANAGEMENT: PROMOTING HARM REDUCTION THROUGH CONCERTED EFFORTS

***Vitalis Chukwuemeka Echebiri, BMLS, AIMLS, MPH****
Department of Chemical Pathology,
National Hospital Abuja, Garki, Abuja

## ABSTRACT

This chapter examines the risk posed by the increasing waste generation all over the world, and proposes harm reduction through global concerted efforts. Industrial revolution and sustained urban growth have resulted in massive generation of various kinds of wastes. Sanitary conditions have therefore continued to worsen, leading to population harm and painful reduction in the overall quality of life due to breeding of diseases and outbreaks. Most often, the unexpected rise in the number of disease cases overwhelms the available health facilities leading to preventable deaths. Although legislations to manage wastes abound in various countries, the rate of generation outweighs the capacity to manage these wastes. Regrettably, some countries generate very toxic wastes which are illegally transported to unsuspecting countries for

* Email: echetalys@yahoo.com.

disposal, not minding the harm these will cause the population in those countries. This action undermines the global campaign for good health for all, and therefore calls for global commitment toward a better and safer waste management mechanism geared toward promoting cleaner and healthier environment with concomitant harm reduction to the global population.

## INTRODUCTION

Public health as an organ of health system has strived to maintain its relevance over the years amidst unstable global conditions. Maintaining its tripartite objective of promoting health, preventing diseases and prolonging life [1] is a major hurdle especially as these functions have to depend on the combined efforts of the society. Achieving these objectives becomes difficult considering the complexity of the society comprising varying strata of individuals with different levels of education, enlightenment, awareness, cultural disposition and personality perception. Advancing the course of public health to create the desired impact therefore requires bringing all components of the society to a minimum acceptable standard of practice at both individual and collective level that will ensure an overall safety of the society. This in turn depends on the environmental condition upon which the society operates. Maintaining a healthy environment translates directly to overall public health. This is because the environment plays a major role in the disease transmission chain [2]. With regard to the epidemiological triad [3], transmission of an infection can only occur in an environment favorable to both the disease vector and the causative organism (pathogen). Other agents such as solid, liquid and gaseous substances that elicit ill health are also borne by the environment. Creating a safe and clean environment becomes a necessity toward achieving good health in the society. The need therefore arises to evolve proper waste management system as a way of creating conducive environment for good health and high quality of life.

Waste management has become a major concern for nations, municipalities, corporations, and individuals around the world [4], and the global community at large [5] as a result of accelerated generation of wastes arising from increasing population growth, booming economy, rapid urbanization and the rise in community living standards [6]. The primary purposes of waste management strategies are to address the health, environmental, aesthetic, land-use, resource, and economic concerns associated with improper disposal of waste [7,4,5].

## Definition/Categorization of Wastes

Wastes are classified as either controlled or non-controlled wastes based on the UK Environment Agency criteria [8]. Controlled wastes comprise wastes generated from households (municipal wastes), and activities such as commercial, industrial, construction and demolition. Non-controlled wastes comprise wastes arising from activities such as agricultural, mining, dredging operations and quarrying. Municipal wastes are made up of several components which include food, garden wastes, papers, cardboard, glass, metals, plastics and textiles. They could also arise from commercial and industrial activities; however, substantial quantities of chemical and mineral wastes are produced in addition, depending on the sector. Wastes generated from agricultural activities include primarily slurry, farmyard manure, and significant amounts of straw, silage effluent, vegetables and cereal residues. Certain wastes are classified as hazardous or toxic because of their intrinsic harmful nature. An example of hazardous waste is toxic explosive. The three largest forms of wastes in this group are oils and oily wastes, construction and demolition waste and asbestos, and wastes from organic chemical processes [9].

Hospital wastes constitute another category of wastes. Hospitals generate a small proportion of wastes classified as infectious and hazardous [10], but a greater percentage of wastes generated in hospitals (about 85%) are classified as general wastes with similar characteristics as municipal wastes [11]. Basically hospital wastes are classified into seven categories namely: (i) general waste: this has similar form as the common household wastes. This type of waste is non-hazardous and non-infectious in nature. Examples are papers, packaging materials, plastics and wrappers; (ii) pathologic waste: this comprises tissues, organs, body parts, blood and other body fluids. Pathogenic waste could be hazardous and infectious in nature; (iii) infectious waste: this type of waste is both hazardous and infectious and contains sufficient amount of pathogens that can cause diseases. Examples are wastes from patients having infectious diseases, culture and stocks of infectious organisms from laboratories, surgical wastes etc; (iv) Sharps: these are wastes that can cause physical harm like cut and puncture to a person handling them. They could be infectious depending on their source. Examples are needles, scalpels, surgical blades, injection ampoules and broken glasses; (v) Pharmaceutical wastes: these include pharmaceutical products like medicines and chemicals which are spilled, expired or contaminated. They are hazardous in nature; (vi) Chemical wastes: these include solid, liquid and gaseous chemicals used for various purposes such as disinfection and cleaning; (vii) Radioactive wastes: these consist of solid, liquid and gaseous materials that are contaminated with radioactive substances generated from in-vitro analysis of body tissues and fluids, body organ imaging and tumour localization and therapeutic procedures [10,11].

Biomedical wastes constitute another distinct group in the categorization of wastes. They include solid and liquid products generated from diagnostic procedures, treatment, immunization, research, testing of biologicals and wastes from humans and animals. Biomedical wastes are generally infectious and hazardous [12].

## Effects of Wastes on Public Health

The public health effects of wastes have been comprehensively reviewed in a study by Vrijheid [13]. The health problems investigated include respiratory symptoms, skin irritation, nose and eyes irritation, gastrointestinal disorders, allergies, fatigue, headaches and psychological problems. There is an assumption that an evaluation of the relationships between these symptoms is confounded by public perception of risk, odour, stress, nuisance associated with the site, and information bias (especially recall). A survey carried out in this regard showed that residents who expressed worries about pollution reported more symptoms than those who were indifferent, in both the exposed and control areas [14]. However, two studies in the US found an increased frequency of cancers in counties that have hazardous waste sites [15,16], especially oesophageal, stomach, colon and rectal cancers. As important as these studies appear, they are limited by lack of chemical release data. Conversely, studies [17,18] on the Love Canal site found no increase in the frequency of cancer rates or the frequency of chromosomal changes. Whereas there were reports of increased incidence of cancer among people living near the Miron Quarry site, which is the third largest in North America, particularly cancers of the liver, kidney, pancreas and non-Hodgkin's lymphomas [19,20]. Once again these studies were not robust as measurements of exposure were not carried out, and the periods of exposure were relatively short.

The effects on human reproduction associated with landfilled sites have been extensively studied. These include low birth weight (less than 2500 g), fetal and infant mortality, spontaneous abortion, and occurrences of birth defects. Two different studies [21,22] reported increased frequency of low birth weight in the populations around the Love Canal site, especially during the periods of active dumping (1940–1953) and among house owners from 1965 to 1978. This trend in the proportion of low birth weight babies was also observed among people residing within 1 km radius of the Lipari Landfill in New Jersey, particularly between 1971 and 1975 during which heavy pollution of streams and a nearby lake occurred as a result of leaching from the site [23]. These patterns in low birth weight and neonatal deaths were observed at a large hazardous waste disposal site in California corresponding closely with time and quantities of dumping, and significantly, lower birth weights were recorded in exposed areas than control areas during the periods of heaviest dumping [24]. The results of studies of congenital malformations are not as convincing as those of low birth weight. Two studies of multiple site in the US were at variance; the first study [25] reported a small increase of about 1.5-folds in heart and circulatory malformations but no increased risk for other malformations, while the second study [26] found no association, although the questionnaire used to collect data recorded a relatively poor response of about 63%, and how congenital malformations were defined was very unclear. However, a study in the UK [27] reported significantly elevated risks for several defects, including neural tube defects, abdominal wall defects, hypospadias and epispadias, and possibly there was a tendency for a higher risk in the incidence of these defects in the period prior to opening of a landfill site compared with after the opening. A similar finding was reported among people residing near the Welsh landfill of Nant-y-Gwyddon with the risk of congenital malformation rates nearly doubled in exposed areas both before and after the opening of the site. However, in four cases, it was observed that there was an exponential increase of as much as nine-folds in gastroschisis, after opening of the site [28]. A study of 21 European hazardous waste sites found that people living within 3 km of a site had significantly high risk of congenital anomaly, with a fairly proportionate decrease in risk as the distance away from the sites increased. There were higher risks of neural-tube defects, malformations of the cardiac septa and anomalies of great arteries and veins than other abnormalities [29]. The same group of researchers in another study [30] found similar increases in chromosomal abnormalities, even after adjusting for maternal age. All the studies of congenital malformations around dumping waste sites generally used residential proximity as a measure of exposure. A similar study conducted in New York State attempted to investigate associations with off-site migration of chemicals and certain categories of chemicals present at the sites [31]. It was found that a statistically significant risk of congenital malformation associated with maternal proximity to a site was small (about 12%), which increased with off-site chemical leaks. Significant associations in musculoskeletal system defects were observed for pesticides filled sites; metals and solvents caused nervous system defects, while plastics caused chromosomal abnormalities.

## Waste Utilization

Before the period of industrial revolution, resources were relatively scarce. Anything valuable in the waste stream was ransacked, and consumer items were recovered for reuse, and damaged ones were repaired rather than been discarded and allowed to be destroyed in the waste stream [5]. This situation re-emerged as cities grew in size with more people to cater for during the industrial revolution. Once again the resource value of wastes rose again, and dustbin and garbage pickers scavenged for valuable items from the waste streams for reuse and selling. This activity is still been practiced today in many developing countries. However, recycling rates dropped from the high levels recorded during the pre-industrial times to single digits by the 1970s [5]. This period was characterized by tremendous rise in consumption, aggressive marketing of commodities, and very low regard for resource conservation.

In order to boost production and sustain the high level of consumption, there was urgent need to improve soil quality to support food production. This resulted in the mobilization of organic wastes as manure. Organic wastes have increasingly found usage in agriculture for the purpose of improving the soil physical and chemical properties and for nutrient sources for growing crops. The major source of organic wastes for agricultural use is animal wastes, but small amounts of processed materials, industrial wastes and municipal wastes are also been used. However, in the last four decades, environmental regulations on the use of organic wastes as manure have resulted in more manure treatment for land use [32]. Reuse of wastes is regarded as a conservative way of utilizing natural resources. Currently, the Taiwan's Environmental Protection Administration encourages the reuse of wastes as a way of resource conservation and pollution prevention, a measure which has reduced waste treatment and disposal costs, while substantially improving productivity [33]. Waste reuse has been exploited in biodiesel production whereby disposable cooking oil containing large quantities of free fatty acids is utilized and catalytically treated to produce biodiesel. The physical and chemical properties of biodiesel produced in this way were found to be of good quality, and satisfied the requirement of relevant international standards [34]. The biodiesel produced through this technique gave a high engine performance with low emission following further refining [34]

## Waste Management Strategies

Waste Management is a complex venture that is carried out in a definite pattern if adequate sanitation and public health are to be given the required attention. Managing wastes depends on the category and characteristics of the wastes. For waste management to be effective, the waste should be managed at every step, from acquisition to final disposal. A comprehensive waste management system has the following components: waste survey, segregation, accumulation and storage, transportation, treatment, disposal, and waste minimization.

The steps in waste management are summarized as follows [35,36]:

*Waste survey:* A survey is meant to differentiate and quantify the waste generated, determine the points of generation, the type of waste at every point and the degree of generation and treatment of the waste. The method of waste disposal is decided following this process.

*Waste segregation:* This entails sorting different kinds of wastes in different coded bags or containers at the point of generation. This practice reduces the bulk of hazardous and infectious wastes and reduces treatment costs as well. Segregation essentially helps to create warning signal about the dangers of wastes meant for disposal, thereby preventing potential harm and infection to the public.

*Waste accumulation and storage:* This process takes place between points of waste generation and site of waste treatment and disposal. Accumulation of wastes means temporarily gathering of wastes in small quantities close to the point of generation, while waste storage entails aggregating wastes in large quantities at bigger collection points for longer periods. An offsite aggregation of waste is regarded as storage. To control and contain spills, storage site or container should be made to have a leak proof floor that will be able to hold enough fluids that could be generated from the degradation of the stored wastes. The storage sites should be easy to clean as well, and should be cleaned and disinfected at regular intervals. Storage sites should be sited close to waste treatment points. Most importantly, storage zones should be clearly labeled with caution signs for proper identification.

*Waste transportation:* This process entails transporting wastes from points of generation to points of accumulation and storage for proper treatment and storage before the final disposal.

*Waste treatment:* Treatment of waste is carried out to modify it through disinfection and decontamination. This practice makes wastes less hazardous and less infectious, and safer for transportation, storage and final disposal.

*Waste disposal:* The methods of waste disposal vary according to handling volume, cost, and impacts on the environment. Some of the available disposal methods include thermal methods (low and high), incineration, autoclaving, microwaving, chemical methods, ionizing radiation process and deep burial. Incineration and autoclaving are considered traditional methods. A solar heating system for disinfecting infectious wastes in economically less developed countries has been developed [37]. This method causes a considerable reduction in the amount of viable bacteria. Untreated wastes are usually disposed off in sanitary landfills. However, this practice is associated with health hazards as highlighted earlier in this chapter.

*Waste minimization:* General waste, whether solid or liquid does not require treatment prior to disposal, whereas all hazardous and infectious wastes must first be treated before disposal to ensure public safety. The cost of disposal of hazardous and infectious wastes may be ten times the cost of disposing general wastes. It therefore follows that any step taken to reduce the quantities of hazardous and infectious wastes generated will give a concomitant reduction in the cost of disposal [38].

*Cost of waste management:* The construction, operation and maintenance of waste management systems are cost intensive, and therefore require a substantial amount of money. If possible waste management should be placed in separate line of state's budget. These costs should be given adequate consideration before a waste management facility is sited. However, it is possible to reduce cost through on-site treatment methods in large facilities. An effective waste management system should be able to provide regular supply of color coded bags, daily collection, safe transportation to the treatment facilities and final disposal with suitable technology [39].

## Dumping of Hazardous/Toxic and Infectious Wastes Across International Boundaries

The past two decades witnessed a tremendous increase in generation and trans-boundary movements of hazardous/toxic wastes [40]. The disposal of these wastes has also become a major issue of environmental justice. It is estimated that about 400 million metric tons of hazardous/toxic waste was generated worldwide in 1990 alone. More than ninety per cent of this volume of waste was generated in Europe [40]. Incidentally, disposal facilities for disposing of these hazardous wastes have become very scarce and more costly in the highly industrialized countries of Europe and America. This situation stimulated the need to find an easier and less costly way of disposing of these wastes. This puts a heavy burden on countries that lack the capacity to handle the wastes in a proper way that will preserve the safety of the environment. Unfortunately, the easy way out is to export these wastes to the developing countries for dumping. This dehumanizing practice of exporting hazardous wastes for disposal in the developing countries has been described as environmental injustice or environmental racism on a global scale [41]. It also portrays socioeconomic inequality of some kind, particularly as these hazardous/toxic wastes find their way into disadvantaged communities where the disposal facilities are usually sited [41]. What makes this practice of international exportation of hazardous wastes and the sitting of disposal facilities in disadvantaged communities within the developing countries unjust and unfair is that the poor communities are made to bear the burden of industrialization without necessarily enjoying any of the benefits.

Nigeria witnessed one of the earliest cases of illegal dumping. In what was supposed to be a genuine business transaction that granted an Italian national working in Nigeria a product import license, what eventually transpired was an illegal deal whereby the supposed consumer products were substituted with shipments of several thousand tons of highly toxic and carcinogenic radioactive wastes, together with 150 tons of polychlorinated biphenyls. An estimated 3,800 tons of these wastes were dumped at a site around Koko ports. Investigations revealed that when the fraud was eventually discovered and the Italian company was forced to evacuate the toxic waste shipments, many vessels containing these wastes had already been badly damaged and leaked. The harmful nature of these toxic wastes manifested among workers who packed the vessels into containers for re-shipment to Italy. Some of them suffered severe chemical burns, and were hospitalized; while one of them got paralyzed. The land within 500 meters radius of the dump site was declared unsafe and there have been public health concerns about surface and groundwater contamination even after the waste was evacuated [42].

After what happened in Nigeria, the international toxic waste dumping took a new dimension; assuming an economic undertone. In 1988, an offer of $600 million dollar was made to Guinea-Bissau, an amount four folds its gross national product, to dispose of 15 million tons of toxic wastes over a period of five years. The contract suffered a setback due to public concern within Guinea-Bissau [42]. During the same period of 1980s, other African countries which included Namibia, Guinea, Haiti and Sierra Leone were made similar offer [42]. Unfortunately, dumping took place in some cases with the connivance of the governments or government officials in the affected countries, while in other cases it was carried out as an illegal operation [42]. The economic incentives for dumping of hazardous wastes in developing countries are always attractive and irresistible as a result of poverty.

The perceived environmental hazards that could occur from dumping of hazardous waste in developing countries attracted international attention for the first time in the late 1980's, when several cases of dumping in Africa were reported [40]. Notwithstanding, developing countries remained vulnerable to international dumping because they provide a disposal option at prices that are often a meager fraction of the actual cost in the developed countries. One study [40] in the late 1980's, revealed that the average disposal costs for 1 ton of hazardous wastes in the developed countries ranged between $100 USD and $2,000 USD, while it costs between a paltry $2.50 USD and $50 USD to dispose of the same quantity of waste in Africa [40]. The lower costs of waste disposal in the developing countries generally portray lack of environmental standards, less stringent laws and absence of public opposition due to lack of information and enlightenment about the potential dangers involved [40]. Without regulation developing countries increasingly continued to be vulnerable, since like a downhill flow of water, hazardous wastes will always be disposed of along the path of least resistance and least cost [43]. This therefore called for international regulation against international dumping of hazardous and toxic wastes. As industrialized countries accepted to acknowledge the dangers of unsafe and improper disposal of hazardous wastes, more stringent environmental and safety measures were therefore put in place. Consequently, disposal of hazardous/toxic wastes became extremely difficult and expensive.

## Policy Issues on Waste Management

Production of wastes in large quantities is as old as human community. As human beings started forming settlement around 10,000 BC, waste production on a large scale became inevitable due to increase in consumption, proportionate to rising population [44]. The need to checkmate the rising waste production evoked public health concerns. Apart from maintaining environmental safety and aesthetics, developing a waste management system became necessary due to dwindling resources [45-47,5,44]. Before the modern waste management, communities merely bury generated wastes away from their settlements or dump in nearby rivers. However, with a rise in population densities these practices became ineffective in preventing foul smell and diseases [5]. Unfortunately, uncontrolled generation of wastes and poor disposal system led to communities co-habiting with the accumulated wastes.

Expansion of cities in the Europe and America as a result of industrial revolution necessitated a revolution in waste management for both human and environmental safety. Interestingly, a milestone in waste management was recorded between 1790 and 1850 in London, where collection of household ashes generated from coal used in cooking became a big business owing to very high demand of ashes as raw material for bricks' making [5]. The actual sanitary revolution started in London in the twilight of the 1830s with the establishment of Sanitation Commission, which established the first clear association between disease and poor sanitary conditions. Based on this premise government's interest in public health became stronger, leading to a leap in waste management system backed by legislation. Government's involvement brought about greater investment in infrastructure and policy enforcement. Between 1848 and 1875 Public Health Acts were enacted, requiring households to dispose of their wastes in moveable receptacles, which were emptied weekly by the local authorities. Subsequently, other countries in Europe enacted and implemented similar legislations [5].

Waste disposal became a political agenda in the industrialized countries through the industrial movement of 1960s and 1970s [5,49]. which significantly elicited a shift in policymakers' perspectives on how to approach waste management [50]. Further legislations to address all forms of wastes were enacted with an initial objective of eliminating uncontrolled disposal. Subsequent legislations increasingly emphasized environmental standards to reduce the contamination of air, land, and water [5]. The environmental movement acted as a primary driver of the policy stages from the 1970s onwards [5]. Waste Management policy from the 1970s to mid-1980s focused on controlling waste, and promoted measures such as the daily covering and compacting of landfills and overhauling of incinerators in order to control dust. Subsequent policy formulations emerged in the 1980s, and continued till date, focus on gradual upgrading of technical standards, beginning with landfill gases and control of leaching, incinerator gas and dioxin reduction, and now traversing to odour control for composting facilities and anaerobic digesters [5]. In the 1990s, integrative policy took the front burner when it was evident that canvassing for ever increasing environmental protection was not enough. An integrative regulatory approach was therefore necessary if environmental protection was to be realized as it was meant to incorporate the technical and environmental components with political, social, financial, economic, and institutional elements of waste management [50,51,5].

With other macroeconomic problems competing for limited resources, it become necessary for the public process of waste management goal formulation to take a democratic dimension to determine the actual needs of the citizens, and set priorities for limited municipal resources in a fair manner. Essentially, the failure of most waste management systems in the developing countries is caused by policy weaknesses, as inadequate formulation and implementation of realistic policies are commonplace [52]. The developed countries in contrast handle their waste management issues by formulating effective and functional policy measures.

An effective waste management system must have clearly defined roles and legal responsibilities of institutions and government bodies to prevent controversies, ineffectiveness, inaction, and unstable political framework [53]. Even when regulatory and legislative frameworks exist, governments with weak institutional structures are easily overwhelmed by increasing demands for waste management as urban populations expand [54, 55,52). Good governance of waste management system therefore requires the participation and collaboration of all relevant parties, including government, non-governmental organizations (NGOs), the private sector and community associations [52].

## Advancing Regulatory Framework for National and International Waste Management

In the last couple of years the need to protect the environment has been extended to the protection of endangered communities. This form of non-traditional environmentalism is known as environmental justice or environmental racism [41]. The movement has its roots in the US, and received national recognition in 1982 following the jailing of over 500 protesters who opposed the siting of a landfill in Warren County, North Carolina. The demonstration was sparked off by a decision to include approximately 330,000 cubic yards of polychlorinated biphenyl (PCB) contaminated soil in landfill. After this incident, many studies in the US established a correlation between race, socio-economic status and the location of hazardous waste facilities [41]. Consequently, it became obvious that the success of any waste management system depends largely on the social components and community priorities [56, 57,55,58,59]. Factors such as public acceptance, changing value systems, public participation in planning and implementation stages, and consumer behavior are comparatively as important as the technical and economic aspects of waste management [56]. An effective waste management system must fully integrate local authorities and the public sphere, and transcend beyond traditional consultative methods that require expert solution prior to public involvement [7,58]. The key components for the success of waste management system include public participation and empowerment, decision transparency, networking, co-operation, communication, accessibility of information and collective action [56,60].

The Basel Convention on the Control of trans-boundary movements of hazardous wastes and their disposal is one major important measure taken in recent times toward international regulation of hazardous/toxic waste [61]. Basel Convention which came into being in 1992 was negotiated in 1989 following international concerns about exports of hazardous wastes to developing countries. Although, the Basel Convention is not a direct concept of environmental justice; its underlying principles provide practical structures for protection of human health and the environment in the developing countries. The ratification of the Basel Convention was objectively meant to achieve one of the overall targets of achieving sustainable environmental development as listed in Agenda 21 [40]. Over one hundred countries have so far accepted and ratified the Convention. It is, however, worrisome to clarify that the initial ideology of the Basel Convention was not to place a ban on trans-boundary movements of hazardous waste; rather it undertakes to control and minimize the movement of wastes, so that transportation and disposal of the wastes are carried out in a manner that will ensure human and environmental safety [61]. This ideology is a subtle way of paying lip service to a grievous human right violation on a matter affecting public health especially in the developing countries, and invariably encouraging continued trans-boundary movement of hazardous/toxic wastes across international borders. Regrettably, since after the Basel Convention was negotiated and ratified it has not come into force nor has it been amended to impose a ban on export of hazardous wastes from European to non-European countries [61].

## Challenges of Waste Management System

Waste management system is affected by a lot of factors, just like every other system. These challenges encompass all aspects of waste management system. Waste generation as a matter of fact is influenced by family size, level of education and income level [62]. On the other hand, attitudes of households in relation to separation of wastes are usually affected by the active support and investment of a real estate company, involvement of community residential committees for public participation [63]; fee for collection service based on the volume or weight of waste [64]; Gender, peer influence, land size, location of household and membership of environmental organization [65]. The collection, transfer and transportation of wastes are affected by lack of information about collection schedule, poor route planning and improper bin collection systems, poorly developed, or insufficient infrastructure, bad and poor road network and limited number of vehicles for waste collection [66,67,7]. It is, however, possible to achieve an effective and inexpensive waste collection services through organizing the informal sector and promoting micro-enterprises participation [68].

In the area of waste treatment, lack of knowledge of treatment systems by authorities is a major factor affecting this process [69]. Collection and storage of wastes normally precede waste treatment. These processes require adhering to proper waste disposal practices by households, but analysis has shown that households' waste disposal decision making are affected by supply of waste facilities [70]. Limited supply of waste bins and long distance to these bins increase the possibility of open and roadside dumping of wastes relative to the use of communal waste bins. In any case, insufficient financial resources and absence of legislation are strong factors that could impair safe disposal of wastes even in well equipped and engineered landfills [71].

With regard to recycling of wastes, there are supporting arguments that high rates of recovery are associated with tipping fees at the disposal site [72]; and high disposal pricing promotes better recovery and beneficial reuse of wastes [73]. As a matter of fact, some communities have been shown to have strong recycling habit due to social influences, altruistic and regulatory factors

[74]. Comparatively, people who often go to the bins to dispose of general refuse are more likely to recycle some items at home, and in most cases, as the distance to the bins decreases, the rate of recovery and recycling of items from wastes to be disposed of increases. In practical terms, recycling rates can be grossly improved if the government develops or encourages the development of markets for recycled materials as well as promoting professionalism in companies involved in recycling [75]. Other factors that can improve recycling culture include, providing adequate financial support for recycling projects and infrastructures, encouraging development of many recycling companies; establishment of drop-off and buy back centers; encouraging active participation of the informal sector, provision of right technologies and reliable data [76,7,77-79].

Waste management system to a large extent is driven by huge financial cost if service provision is to be sustained [68]. The absence of financial support, limited resources, users' unwillingness to pay for the service and lack of proper use of economic instruments could pose serious hindrance to the delivery of proper waste management services [62]. The involvement of the private sector with adequate legal framework could improve the efficiency of the system [78]. It is erroneously assumed that waste management is the sole responsibility of local authorities, and that the public is not expected to contribute [80]; however, studies have shown that the operational efficiency of waste management depends on active participation of both the municipal agency and the citizens [78]. Therefore, people's participation in decision making and community awareness are important toward the success of waste management [67,78]. While emphasizing the need to give due consideration to all factors affecting waste management system as the first step toward proffering an effective solution, it is important to acknowledge that waste disposal workers are accorded low social status [80]. Politicians give low priority to waste disposal activities compared to other municipal activities as a result of which very few trained and skilled personnel are available [67,78]. This situation leads to low motivation among the waste disposal employees, causing delays in proper waste treatment and disposal. According waste disposal workers due recognition with good remuneration and regular training will go a long way in enhancing effective waste management system. Factors that support municipal authorities and strategic plans for waste management system that allow regular monitoring and evaluation should be adopted [81,82]. Overall, adequate legal framework can contribute positively to the development of integrated waste management system [82], while the absence of satisfactory policies [79] and weak regulations [83] could be detrimental to it.

## Conclusion

The role of public health is unequivocally central to healthy living and general wellbeing of the world's population. Incidentally, this role cannot be administered in a vacuum. The environment inevitably provides the right platform for public health to operate. Invariably, neglecting the environment translates to treating a disease without understanding its cause and natural history. The consequence will be a serious epidemic that will only be contained by divine intervention. Maintaining a healthy environment therefore is the first step toward preventing diseases, which translates directly to promoting health and ultimately prolonging life. Waste management is indeed a sure way of creating a safe and healthy environment.

Over the years, waste management has become increasingly difficult as a result of massive generation of wastes arising from population growth and industrial revolution. Some of these wastes being hazardous and toxic have caused serious harm to public health leading to various kinds of diseases and preventable deaths. Disposing of these wastes is now a major concern to public health. As the cost of disposal continues to rise in the developed countries, the developing countries have become the target for dumping at a very meager cost, and grave consequence to public health. Although, legislations abound within national and international circles to control the disposal of wastes to protect the environment and public health, unfortunately, some of these legislations are inactive or inoperative. The Basel Convention is an international legislation meant to control and minimize the trans-boundary movement of wastes. The failure of this legislation to place a ban on trans-boundary movements of hazardous wastes is a subtle way of paying lip service to a grievous human right violation on a matter affecting public health especially in the developing countries, and invariably encouraging continued trans-boundary movement of hazardous/toxic wastes across international borders. It is therefore necessary to evolve a system that will enhance immediate recycling and disposal of wastes as soon as they are generated. A pragmatic approach to an effective waste management system will be the application of an integrative approach involving all the stakeholders such as the government, non-governmental organizations (NGOs), the private sector and community associations who are involved in every aspect of waste management. According waste disposal workers due recognition with good remuneration and regular training will go a long way toward enhancing prompt and proper waste disposal. Factors that support municipal authorities and strategic plans for waste management system that allow regular monitoring and evaluation should be adopted. Overall, adequate legal framework, satisfactory policies and strong regulations with binding force will contribute positively to the development of integrated waste management system. However, a global commitment to a better and safer waste management system is strongly required toward promoting safer and healthier environment with a concomitant harm reduction to the global population.

## REFERENCES


[1] Institute of Medicine. *The Future of Public Health.* Washington: National Academies Press, 1988.

[2] Bailey, L; Vardulaki, K; Langham, J; Chandramohan, D. *Introduction to Epidemiology.* London: Open University Press, 2005.

[3] Merrill, RM. Introduction to Epidemiology (6$^{th}$ ed.). Burlington, MA: Jones & Bartlett Learning, 2013; 6-12.

[4] Nemerow, NL. *Environmental Engineering: Environmental Health and Safety for Municipal Infrastructure, Land Use and Planning, and Industry* (6$^{th}$ ed.). Hoboken, N.J: Wiley, 2009.

[5] Wilson, DC. Development drivers for waste management. *Waste Management & Research* 2007; 3: 198–207.

[6] Minghua, Z; Xiumin, F; Rovetta, A; Qichang, H; Vicentini, F; Bingkai, L; Giusti, A; Yi, L. Municipal solid waste management in Pudong New Area, China. *Journal of Waste Management* 2009; 29: 1227–1233.

[7] Henry, RK.; Yongsheng, Z; Jun, D. Municipal solid waste management challenges in developing countries – Kenyan case study. *Waste Management* 2006; 1: 92–100.

[8] Environment Agency. Waste Statistics for England and Wales 1998–99. London: Environment Agency, 1998.

[9] Rushton, L. Health hazards and waste management. *British Medical Bulletin* 2003; 1: 183-197.

[10] Tsakona, M; Anagnostopoulou, E; Gidarakos, E. Hospital waste management and toxicity evaluation: a case study. *Waste Management* 2007; 27: 912-920.

[11] Chaerui, M; Tanaka, M; Shekdar, AV. A system dynamic approach for hospital waste management. *Waste Management* 2008; 2: 442-449.

[12] Chandra, H. Hospital Waste: An Environmental Hazard and Its Management. *Archives* 1999; 5: 3.

[13] Vrijheid, M. Health effects of residence near hazardous waste landfill sites: a review of epidemiologic literature. *Environ Health Perspect,* 2000; 108: 101–12.

[14] Ozonoff D; Colten ME; Cupples A; Heeren T; Schatzkin A; Mangione T; Dresner M; Colton T. Health problems reported by residents of a neighbourhood contaminated by a hazardous waste facility. *Am J Ind Med* 1987; 11: 581–97.

[15] Najem, GR; Louria, DB; Lavenhar, MA; Feuerman, M. Clusters of cancer mortality in New Jersey municipalities: with special reference to chemical toxic waste disposal sites and per capita income. *Int J Epidemiol* 1983; 12: 276–88.

[16] Griffith, J; Duncan, R; Riggan, W; Peloma, A. Cancer mortality in US counties with hazardous waste sites and ground water pollution. *Arch Environ Health* 1989; 44: 69–74.

[17] Janerich DT; Burnett WS; Feck G; Hoff M; Nasca P; Polednak AP; Greenwald P;Vianna N. Cancer incidence in the Love Canal area. *Science* 1981; 212: 1404–7.

[18] Heath, CW; Nadel, MR; Zack, MM; Chen, ATL; Bender, MA; Preston, RJ. Cytogenetic findings in persons living near the Love Canal. *JAMA* 1984; 251: 1217–9.

[19] Goldberg, MS; Al-Homsi, N; Goulet, L; Riberdy, H. Incidence of cancer among persons living near a municipal solid waste landfill site in Montreal, Quebec. *Arch Environ Health* 1995; 50: 416–24.

[20] Goldberg, MS; DeWar, R; Desy, M; Riberdy, H. Risk of developing cancer relative to living near a municipal solid waste landfill site in Montreal, Quebec, Canada. *Arch Environ Health* 1999; 54: 291–6.

[21] Vianna, NJ; Polan, AK. Incidence of low birthweight among Love Canal residents. *Science* 1984; 226: 1217–9.

[22] Goldman, LR; Paigen, B; Magnant, MM; Highland, JH. Low birthweight, prematurity and birth defects in children living near the hazardous waste site, Love Canal. *Hazard Waste Hazard Mater* 1985; 2: 209–23.

[23] Berry, M; Bove, F. Birthweight reduction association with residence near a hazardous waste landfill. *Environ Health Perspect* 1997; 105: 856–61.

[24] Kharazi, M; Von Behren, J; Smith, M; Lomas, T; Armstrong, M; Broadwin, R; Blake E; McLaughlin B; Worstell G; Goldman L. A community based study of adverse pregnancy outcomes near a large hazardous waste landfill in California. *Toxicol Ind Health* 1997; 13: 299–310.

[25] Shaw, GM; Schulman, J; Frisch, JD; Cummins, SK; Harris, JA. Congenital malformations and birthweight in areas with potential environmental contamination. *Arch Environ Health* 1992; 47: 147–54.

[26] Sosniak, WA; Kaye, WE; Gomez, TM. Data linkage to explore the risk of low birthweight associated with maternal proximity to hazardous waste sites from the National Priorities list. *Arch Environ Health* 1994; 49: 251–5.

[27] Elliott, P; Briggs, D; Morris, S; de Hoogh, C; Hurt, C; Jensen, TK.; Maitland I, Richardson S, Wakefield J, Jarup L. Risk of adverse outcomes in populations living near landfill sites. *BMJ* 2001; 363–368.

[28] Fielder, HMP; Poon-King, C; Palmer, SR; Coleman, G. Assessment of the impact on health of residents living near the Nant-y-Gwyddon landfill site: Retrospective analysis. *BMJ* 2000; 320: 19–23.

[29] Dolk, H; Vrijheid, M; Armstrong, B; Abramsky, L; Bianchi, F; Garne, E; Nelen V; Robert E; Scott JE; Stone D; Tenconi R. Risk of congenital anomalies near hazardous-waste landfill sites in Europe: the EUROHAZCON study. *Lancet* 1998; 352: 423–427

[30] Vrijheid M; Dolk H; Armstrong B; Abramsky L; Bianchi F; Fazarinc I; Garne E; Ide R; Nelen V; Robert E; Scott JE; Stone D; Tenconi R. Chromosomal congenital anomalies and residence near hazardous waste landfill sites. *Lancet* 2002; 359: 320–322.

[31] Geshwind, SA; Stowijk, JAJ; Bracken, M; Fitzgerald E; Stark A; Olsen C; Melius J. Risk of congenital malformations associated with proximity to hazardous waste sites. *Am J Epidemiol* 1992; 135:1197–1207.

[32] Westerman, PW; Bicudo, JR. Management considerations for organic waste use in agriculture. *Bioresource Technology* 2005; 2: 215-221.

[33] Tsai, WT; Chou, YH. Government policies for encouraging industrial waste reuse and pollution prevention in Taiwan. *Journal of Cleaner Production* 2004; 7: 725-736.

[34] Meng, X; Chen, G; Wang, Y. Biodiesel production from waste cooking oil via alkali catalyst and its engine test. *Fuel Processing Technology* 2008; 9: 851-857.

[35] Gordon, JG; Rein, Hardt, PA; Denys, GA. Medical waste management. In: Mayhall CG (ed). *Hospital epidemiology and infection control, (3rd ed.)*. Lippincott: Williams and Wilkins publication, 2004: 1773-85.

[36] Cocchiarella, L; Scott, Deitchman, D; Young, D. Biohazardous waste management: What the physicians need to know. *Arch Fam Med* 2000; 9: 26-9.

[37] Chitnis, V; Chitnis, S; Patil, S; Chitnis, D. Solar disinfection of infectious biomedical waste: A new approach for developing countries. *Lancet* 2003; 362: 1285-1286.

[38] Seymour Block, S. *Disinfection, sterilization and preservation, (5 th ed.)*. Lippincott: Williams and Wilkins publication, 2001.

[39] Rao, SK; Ranyal, RK; Bhatia, SS; Sharma, VR. Biomedical waste management: An infrastructural survey of hospitals. *MJAFI* 2004; 60: 4.

[40] Kummer, K. *International Management of Hazardous Wastes.* Oxford: Clarendon Press, 1995; 10.

[41] Marbury, HR. "Global Environmental Racism". *Vanderbilt Journal of Transnational Law* 1995; 28: 251-293.

[42] Vir, A. "Toxic Trade with Africa". *Environment, Science & Technology Journal* 1989; 1: 24-25.

[43] Porterfield, S; Weir, D. "The Export of US Toxic Waste". *Nation* 1989; 1: 245-344.

[44] Worrell, WA; Vesilind, PA. *Solid Waste Engineering (2nd ed.)*. Stamford, CT: Cengage Learning, 2012.

[45] Louis, GE. A historical context of municipal solid waste management in the United States. *Waste Management & Research* 2004; 4: 306–322.

[46] Melosi, MV. *Garbage in the Cities: Refuse, Reform, and the Environment, 1880-1980 (1st ed.)*. College Station, Texas: Texas A&M University Press, 1981.

[47] Ponting, C. *A Green History of the World: The Environment and the Collapse of Great Civilizations.* New York: St. Martin's Press, 1991.

[48] Seadon, JK. Sustainable waste management systems. *Journal of Cleaner Production* 2010; 18: 1639–1651.

[49] Wolsink, M. Contested environmental policy infrastructure: socio-political acceptance of renewable energy, water, and waste facilities. *Environmental Impact Assessment Review* 2010; 5: 302–311.

[50] McDougall, F; White, PR; Franke, M; Hindle, P. *Integrated Solid Waste Management: A Lifecycle Inventory* (2nd ed.). Oxford, UK: Blackwell Science, 2001.

[51] van de Klundert, A; Anschutz, J. *Integrated sustainable waste management – the concept: tools for decision-makers. Experiences from the Urban Waste Expertise Programme (1995–2001).* In: Scheinberg, A. (Ed.), Gouda, Urban Waste Expertise Programme. Netherlands: UNDP/ UNCHS/World Bank/SDC, 2001.

[52] Konteh, FH. Urban sanitation and health in the developing world: reminiscing the nineteenth century industrial nations. *Health & Place* 2009; 1: 69–78.

[53] Schübeler, P. Conceptual framework for municipal solid waste management in low-income countries. In: Wehrle, K., Christen, J. (Eds.), St. Gallen Switzerland: UNDP/UNCHS/World Bank/SDC Collaborative Programme on Municipal Solid Waste Management in Low-Income Countries, 1996.

[54] Halla, F; Majani, B. Innovative ways for solid waste management in Dar-Es-Salaam: toward stakeholder partnerships. *Habitat International,* 1999; 3: 351–361.

[55] Hardoy, JE; Mitlin, D; Satterthwaite, D; Hardoy, JE. *Environmental Problems in an Urbanizing World: Finding Solutions for Cities in Africa, Asia, and Latin America.* London, Sterling, VA: Earthscan Publications, 2001.

[56] Carabias, WJV; Winistoerfer, H; Stuecheli, A. Social aspects of public waste management in Switzerland. *Waste Management* 1999; 6: 417–425.

[57] Dijkema, GPJ; Reuter, MA; Verhoef, EV. A new paradigm for waste management. *Waste Management* 2000; 8: 633–638.

[58] Morrissey, AJ; Browne, J. Waste management models and their application to sustainable waste management. *Waste Management* 2004; 3: 297–308.

[59] Petts, J. Municipal waste management: inequities and the role of deliberation. *Risk Analysis* 2000; 6: 821–832.

[60] Zarate, MA; Slotnick, J; Ramos, M. *Capacity building in rural Guatemala by implementing a solid waste management program. Waste Management* 2008; 28: 2542–2551.

[61] Basel Convention on the Control of Transboundary Movements of Hazardous Wastes and Their Disposal, Reproduced in (1989) 28(3) ILM 652.

[62] Sujauddin, M; Huda, MS; Rafiqul Hoque, ATM. Household solid waste characteristics and management in Chittagong, Bangladesh. *Journal of Waste Management* 2008; 28: 1688–1695.

[63] Zhuang, Y; Wu, SW; Wang, YL; Wu, YZ; Chen, YX. Source separation of household waste: a case study in China. *Journal of Waste Management* 2008; 28: 2022–2030.

[64] Scheinberg, A; Spies, S; Simpson, MH; Mol A.P.J. Assessing urban recycling in low-and-middle income countries: Building on modernised mixtures *Habitat International* 2011; 35: 188–198.

[65] Ekere, W; Mugisha, J; Drake, L. Factors influencing waste separation and utilization among households in the Lake Victoria crescent, Uganda. *Journal of Waste Management* 2009; 29: 3047–3051.

[66] Hazra, T; Goel, S. Solid waste management in Kolkata, India: practices and challenges. *Journal of Waste Management* 2009; 29: 470–478.

[67] Moghadam, MRA; Mokhtarani, N; Mokhtarani, B. Municipal solid waste management in Rasht City, Iran. *Journal of Waste Management* 2009; 29: 485–489.

[68] Sharholy, M; Ahmad, K; Vaishya, RC; Gupta, RD. Municipal solid waste characteristics and management in Allahabad, India. *Journal of Waste Management* 2007; 27: 490–496.

[69] Chung, S; Lo, C. Local waste management constraints and waste administrators in China. *Journal of Waste Management* 2008; 28: 272–281.

[70] Tadesse, T; Ruijs, A. Hagos, F. Household waste disposal in Mekelle city, Northern Ethiopia. *Journal of Waste Management* 2008; 28: 2003–2012.

[71] Pokhrel, D; Viraraghavan, T. Municipal solid waste management in Nepal: practices and challenges. *Journal of Waste Management* 2005; 25: 555–562.

[72] Scheinberg, A.*Value added: modes of sustainable recycling in the modernisation of waste management systems.* Netherlands: Wageningen University, 2011.

[73] Scheinberg, A., Wilson, D.C., Rodic, L., 2010. Solid waste management in the World's Cities. UN-Habitat's Third Global Report on the State of Water and Sanitation in the World's Cities. EarthScan, Newcastle-upon-Tyne, UK.

[74] Gonzalez-Torre, PL; Adenso-Diaz, B. Influence of distance on the motivation and frequency of household recycling. *Journal of Waste Management* 2005; 25: 15–23.

[75] Minghua, Z; Xiumin, F: Rovetta, A; Qichang, H; Vicentini, F; Bingkai, L; Giusti, A; Yi, L. Municipal solid waste management in Pudong New Area, China. *Journal of Waste Management* 2009; 29: 1227–1233.

[76] Nissim, I; Shohat, T; Inbar, Y. From dumping to sanitary landfills – Solid waste management in Israel. *Journal of Waste Management* 2005; 25: 323–327.

[77] Matete, N; Trois, C. Towards zero waste in emerging countries – A South African experience. *Journal of Waste Management* 2008; 28: 1480–1492.

[78] Sharholy, M; Ahmad, K; Mahmood, G; Trivedi, RC. Municipal solid waste management in Indian cities. A review. *Journal of Waste Management* 2008; 28: 459–467.

[79] Mrayyan, B; Hamdi, MR. Management approaches to integrated solid waste in industrialized zones in Jordan: a case of Zarqa City. *Journal of Waste Management* 2006; 26: 195–205.

[80] Vidanaarachchi, CK; Yuen, STS; Pilapitiya, S. Municipal solid waste management in the Southern Province of Sri Lanka: problems, issues and challenges. *Journal of Waste Management* 2006; 26: 920–930.

[81] Zurbrügg, C; Drescher, S; Rytz, I; Sinha, M; Enayetullah, I. Decentralised composting in Bangladesh, a win–win situation for all stakeholders. *Resources, Conservation and Recycling* 2005; 43: 281–292.

[82] Asase, M; Yanful, EK; Mensah, M; Stanford, J; Amponsah, S. Comparison of municipal solid waste management systems in Canada and Ghana: a case study of the cities of London, Ontario, and Kumasi, Ghana. *Journal of Waste Management* 2009; 29: 2779–2786.

[83] Seng, B; Kaneko, H; Hirayama, K; Katayama-Hirayama, K. Municipal solid waste management in Phnom Penh, capital city of Cambodia. *Waste Management & Research* 2010; 29: 491–500.

Reviewed by: Obiageli E. *Anigbogu* BSc., MSc.
Department of Physiotherapy, National Hospital Abuja,
Plot 132 Central Business District, P.M.B. 425, Garki,
Abuja – Nigeria

Email: oby2020@yahoo.com

In: Public Health and Harm Reduction
Editor: Meredith B. Morris
ISBN: 978-1-63482-159-9


*Chapter 7*

# HARM REDUCTION FOR PEOPLE WHO INJECT DRUGS THROUGH POINT OF CARE CD4/VIRAL LOAD TESTING IN KENYA

***Kennedy Kinyua, Eva Muluve, Paul Macharia and Helgar Musyoki***
Ministry of Health, National AIDS and STIs Control Programme, Nairobi, Kenya

## ABSTRACT

Global HIV/AIDS disease among people who inject drugs is significant and expanding. Unsafe injecting drug use has resulted in the rapid spread of HIV among drug user networks in countries throughout the world. In Kenya, Injecting drug use (IDU) is an emerging problem which needs urgent attention because of its close association with the rapid spread of HIV which can potentiate local HIV epidemics.

Injecting drug users don't access health care services due to socio-economic factors like absence of empathy, listening, shaming, discrimination, flexibility, lack of disclosure and the cost of health care.

Focused and evidence-based approaches are needed to combat IDU-related HIV in Kenya. In resource-constrained settings like Kenya, it is difficult to do viral load and CD4 cell measurements to start treatment but instead rely on clinical staging. But Studies have shown WHO HIV staging misses many with low CD4.

Researchers have therefore been working to make viral load and CD4 cell testing machines which are cheaper, more accessible and easier to use.

Point of care viral load and CD4 machines could then be introduced into the most remote settings in Kenya to help put more people onto care on the basis of viral load and CD4 counts rather than staging. The new tests would also facilitate the delivery of ART in decentralized settings and possibly improve retention into ART programmes, by speeding the time it takes between when a person gets tested and when he or she goes onto ART.

## INTRODUCTION

The global burden of HIV/AIDS disease among IDUs is significant and expanding. Unsafe injecting drug use has resulted in the rapid spread of HIV among drug user networks in countries throughout the world. There are approximately 16 million injecting drug users worldwide, with approximately 3 million living with HIV. An estimated 10 million injecting drug users are dependent on opiod mostly heroin and are concentrated in Europe, North America, central and south Asia and Australia and more recently, the east coast of Africa (Reid, 2009).

Injecting drug users (IDUs) in sub-Saharan Africa are amongst the most vulnerable populations at risk for HIV infection. Comprising a growing proportion of HIV transmissions in the region, they have been a politically powerless group that lacked access to addiction treatment and HIV prevention and faced persecution from police and communities. Because IDU is emerging in a region where HIV prevalence in the general population is already high, injection can potentiate local HIV epidemics very quickly, given the rapid, explosive nature that is the hallmark of HIV epidemics among IDUs. The World Health Organization (WHO) has determined that needle and syringe exchange programs (NSEPs) among other harm reduction strategies are effective in reducing HIV transmission (UNODC, 2005).

Injecting drug use (IDU) is an emerging problem in Kenya which needs urgent attention because of its close association with the rapid spread of HIV. Currently most of the IDUs are found in large towns of Kenya. A study of 336 heroin users in Nairobi, Kenya found that 44.9% were, or had been, injectors. Of 101 current injectors, 52.5% were HIV positive. This compares with a 13.5% prevalence rate among heroin users who had never injected.

Hepatitis C prevalence also varied dramatically, from 61.4% among current injectors to 3.8% for those who had never injected (Odek-Ogunde et al., 2003).

People who inject drugs in Nairobi town are socially marginalized, discriminated and suffer a disproportionate burden of illness relative to nonusers. PWID in Nairobi town are thought to be overburdened by HIV/AIDS, Hepatitis C and B infections, abscess, diarrhea, skin diseases, injuries from police and mob justice. Quality of health care encounters themselves is influenced by the presence or absence of empathy, listening, shaming, discrimination, flexibility, and disclosure. Rapport development is integral to any clinical interaction, and may be a particularly important element of health care with marginalized PWIDs. The cost of health care is also an expensive as health care is mostly financed by Out-pocket payment in Kenya health facilities. Possession of heroin or injecting materials for Harm reduction is a crime in Nairobi City (Odek-Ogunde et al., 2003).

The 2009 / 10 – 2013 /14 Kenyan strategic plan (KNASP III) highlights the need to prevent new infections among PWID and to “seek innovative ways to reduce HIV transmission.” In 2011, the National Aids Control Council [NACC] announced a plan to provide free HIV prevention and treatment for PWID. Included in the plan are previously disallowed harm reduction methods including needle exchange and neglected services such as psychosocial support for PWID. Methadone is not banned in Kenya but its availability is severely restricted (NACC, 2012).

## Point-of-Care-CD4 Test

CD4 depletion is the hallmark of acquired immune deficiency, and CD4 cell indicate when a person should start antiretroviral treatment. The World Health Organization’s 2010 antiretroviral treatment (ART) guidelines recommend that treatment begin at a CD4 count of 350 cells/mm$^3$ (WHO, 2010).

ART is recommended for all HIV-infected patients. In patients who remain untreated for whatever reason, CD4 counts should be monitored every 3 to 6 months to assess the urgency of ART initiation. A repeat CD4 count 3 months after ART initiation will provide information regarding the magnitude of immune reconstitution. The CD4 count response to ART varies widely, but a poor CD4 response in a patient with viral suppression is rarely an indication for modifying an ARV regimen (NIH, 2014).

The gold standard for CD4 measurement is flow cytometry (Becton Dickinson or Beckman), but this equipment is relatively complex and it requires skilled technicians to perform. Many resource-poor settings simply don't have the infrastructure, human resources or funds to provide convenient access to CD4 cell testing in more remote or rural settings but rely on clinical staging which may miss a large numbers of people with very low CD4 cell counts (Reid, 2011).

Point-of-care CD4 machines can be introduced at most remote settings to help put people on treatment on the basis of their CD4 count rather than clinical staging. Some of these machines incude: the Alere's PIMA CD4 machine, the Daktari CD4 machine and the Zyomyx.Inc CD4 machine. They would facilitate the delivery of ART in decentralized settings and possibly improve retention into ART programmes, by speeding the time it takes between when a person gets tested and when he or she goes onto ART and by reducing loss to follow-up (Reid, 2011).

The impact on life-years saved of using syndromic management, point of care CD4 machine and gold standard flow cytometry would be that initiation on the basis of flow cytometry and POC CD4 would have similar overall costs, but POC CD4 cell tests would result in more life-years saved and thus be more cost-effective. The availability of point-of-care testing would affect retention and the timely initiation of ART. Initiation based upon syndromic management clearly cost the least (almost half of POC), but has the poorest outcomes in terms of life-years saved (Reid, 2011).

## Point of Care Viral Load

Viral load test is described as the number of HIV's genetic material (RNA) per millilitre (copies/ml). It is important indicator of initial and sustained response to ART and should be measured in all HIV-infected patients at entry into care, at initiation of therapy, and on a regular basis thereafter. Pre-treatment viral load level is also an important for an initial ARV regimen. Decreasing viral load following initiation of care is associated with reduced chances of progression to AIDS or death. Therefore, viral load testing is used to measure treatment response. Optimal viral suppression is defined generally as a viral load persistently below the level of detection (HIV RNA <20 to 75 copies/mL, depending on the assay used) (NIH, 2014).

Patients who take ART regularly and don't have resistant virus can get viral suppression in 8 – 24 weeks after ART initiation; rarely, it may take longer. Plasma viral load should be measured before initiation of ART and within 2 to 4 weeks but no later than 8 weeks after treatment initiation or modification. This is to determine: the initial virological response to treatment, appropriate drug combinations and patient adherence to drugs. Repeat viral load measurement should be performed at 4- to 8-week intervals until the level falls below the assay's limit of detection (NIH, 2014).

Viral load is also done within 4 to 8 weeks after changing drug regimen. This is to determine effectiveness of the new drugs. Viral load monitoring should be at every 3 – 4 months or as clinically indicated to confirm continuous viral suppression. Clinicians may extend the interval to 6 months for adherent patients whose viral load has been suppressed for more than 2 years and whose clinical and immunologic status is stable. Otherwise the clinical circumstances will dictate the frequency of viral load testing. Patients who fail to achieve viral suppression should undergo resistance testing to aid in the selection of an alternative regimen (NIH, 2014).

Many sub-Saharan countries have started including viral load testing in their guidelines and that in future, if global guidelines moved, as widely predicted, towards a policy of universal treatment on diagnosis, then viral load testing will become more important than CD4 count in terms of monitoring treatment failure and treatment adherence (Lynch, 2014).

There are several different point-of-care viral load testing machines, some battery-powered, that would make it easy to perform viral load tests in the field. Some include: the Alere Q HIV test, the DRW SAMBA test, the Wave-80 EOSCAPE-HIV test, and the Lumora "BART" test (Lynch, 2014).

Compared to other tests, 63% of the cost of a viral load test is the disposable chemical reagents and other disposables such as filters that form part of any viral load test. These cannot easily be made cheaper. Other costs, however, could be lower with point-of-care testing such as the 11.7% proportion that is due to human resources such as technicians, and the 1.92% that is lab charges. In addition, the 9.6% that is due to quality control might be lower in a self-contained machine (Lynch, 2014).

## CONCLUSION

At present, virological tests can only be performed using expensive equipment in advanced laboratories that can also be problematic to access in resource-limited settings with limited infrastructure.

Intravenous drug users' programmes that can provide point-of-care viral load monitoring would be able to determine whether there is viral load is suppression.

Similarly, CD4 cell count monitoring is supposed to be integral to injecting drug users HIV care and management. Introducing point-of-care CD4 machine would greatly reduce time between testing and initiation of care especially among injecting drug users who access care less often or have no time think about their health.

## REFERENCES

AIDS Control Council KN. The Kenya Analysis of HIV Prevention Response and Modes of HIV 2002.

Grundy CL. *Point-of-care CD4 tests can increase life-years saved with reduced costs compared to flow cytometric CD4 counting.* Sixth International AIDS Society Conference on HIV Pathogenesis, Treatment and Prevention, Rome, abstract MOAD0105, 2011.

Hallett TB, Gregson S, Dube S, Garnett GP. The impact of monitoring HIV patients prior to treatment in resource-poor settings: insights from mathematical modelling. *PLoS Med* 5(3): e53. doi:10.1371/journal.pmed.0050053, 2008.

http://aidsinfo.nih.gov/guidelines/html/1/adult-and-adolescent-arv-guidelines/458/plasma-hiv-1-rna--viral-load--and-cd4-count-monitoring

http://www.ihra.net/what-is-harm-reduction

http://www.unodc.org/pdf/WDR_2005/volume_1_web.pdf *World drug report* volume 1, UNODC 2005.

Huang Y-F Yang JY, Nelson KE, Kuo HS, Lew-Ting CY, Yang CH, Chen CH, Chang FY, Liu HR. Changes in HIV incidence among people who inject drugs in Taiwan following introduction of a harm reduction program: a study of two cohorts. *PLOS Medicine* 11(4): e.1001625, 2014.

Jani I, Sitoe N, Quevedo J, Lehe J, Peter T. *Cost comparison of point-of-care and laboratory CD4 testing in resource-limited settings.* Sixth International AIDS Society Conference on HIV Pathogenesis, Treatment and Prevention, Rome, abstract MOAD0101, 2011.

Larson B, Bistline K, Ndibongo B, Xulu T, Brennan A, Long L, Rosen S, Fox M. *Rapid point-of-care CD4 testing at mobile HIV testing sites to increase linkage to care: an evaluation of a pilot program in South Africa.* Sixth

International AIDS Society Conference on HIV Pathogenesis, Treatment and Prevention, Rome, abstract MOAD0103, 2011.

Lynch S. *Viral load testing – are cost and complexity out-dated arguments?* 2014 Treatment as Prevention Workshop, Vancouver, abstract 5082, 2014

Odek-Ogunde M, Lore W, Owiti FR. *Risky behaviours among injecting drug users in Kenya.* In Proceedings of 14th International Conference on the Reduction of Drug Related Harm. Chiang Mai, Thailand; 2003.

Odek-Ogunde M: *Harm reduction as alternative strategy for prevention of drug abuse and HIV/AIDS in Kenya.* In Proceedings of Third Annual Meeting of Global Research Network Meeting on HIV Prevention in Drug-Using populations. Durban, South Africa; 2000:113-117.

Reid S. Injection drug use, unsafe medical injections, and HIV in Africa: a systematic review. *Harm Reduction Journal* 2009;6:24.

Transmission Study - Kenya National AIDS Countrol Council. In. Nairobi; 2009.

WHO, UNODC, UNAIDS. (2004). Substitution maintenance therapy in the management of opioid dependence and HIV/AIDS prevention: position paper.

World Health Organisation (WHO), *Effectiveness of community-based outreach in preventing HIV/AIDS among injecting drug users.* Geneva, WHO, 2004

World Health Organisation (WHO). Joint United Nations programme on HIV/AIDS (UNAIDS). *Global HIV/AIDS response: epidemic update and health sector progress towards universal access.* Geneva, WHO, 2011

In: Public Health and Harm Reduction
Editor: Meredith B. Morris
ISBN: 978-1-63482-159-9


*Chapter 8*

# MEDICATION ASSISTED THERAPY INTEGRATING MOBILE PHONE TECHNOLOGIES

***Paul Macharia, Eva Muluve and Helgar Musyoki***
Ministry of Health, National AIDS & STIs Control Programme,
Nairobi, Kenya

## ABSTRACT

Accurate harm reduction information is needed if clients are to make informed choices, this can be achieved by strategically improving and availing this information. There are a number of available harm-reduction strategies that are promising have been very successful. The importance of individualizing harm reduction intervention to accommodate the preferences and needs of a targeted person or population cannot be over emphasized. A good harm reduction effort will seek to meet the individual where he or she is at and assist that person in the direction of positive behavior change.

Information and communication technologies could increase access by providing individualized up-to-date harm reduction information to promote health, reduce harm, and support client access to care. Cheaper, efficient and reliable mobile phones avail technological opportunities to offer secure and confidential access to harm reduction information. This could include developing mobile phone applications that would ensure easy access to up-to-date information thus enhancing client literacy.

## Introduction

Harm reduction can be defined as efforts and strategies that practically work to reduce the negative consequences to persons using drugs, it is grounded on the evolving public health and advocacy efforts and due to its effectiveness is increasingly gaining public acceptance as these efforts are neutral on drug legalization (Single, 1995)

Medication Assisted Therapy (MAT) is a harm reduction strategy for People who Inject Drugs (PWIDs) also widely known as opioid substitution therapy (OST) that aims to treat opioid dependence by prescribing medication to replace illicit opioid narcotics such as heroin. Research has shown that MAT is combined with psychosocial support has positive outcomes in reducing drug use, criminal behavior and improved reforming addict's community acceptance and reintegration (WHO, UNODC, UNAIDS, 2004). The World Health Organization (WHO) identifies MAT as one of the nine PWID treatment interventions.

MAT is an intensive program requiring a client's adherence, access to up-to-date and relevant information. Information and Communication Technologies (ICT) could increase access to MAT harm reduction interventions by providing individualized up-to-date harm reduction information to promote health, reduce harm, and support client access to care. In the recent past there are a number of cheaper, efficient and reliable mobile phones availing technological opportunities to offer secure and confidential access to harm reduction information (Tamrat et al., 2012, Phillips et al., 2010). To effectively support MAT intervention for PWIDs, mobile phone technology applications need to be developed and customized to increase information access for client literacy, support and monitor MAT treatment and also geographically observe client trends (Eng et al., 1998).

## Background

Substance abuse causes great harm to the user, their family and the community at large; this is much higher for PWIDs with the harmful effects including physical, mental, psychological and social harms. PWIDs are not only at great risk of HIV/AIDS, hepatitis B and C but also drug overdose related complications including death (Hasanović et al., 2012a, Mehić-Basara et al., 2013). A great burden is also imposed on the society due to the PWIDs criminal, violent and delinquent behavior (Hasanović et al., 2012b).

Medication assisted therapy (MAT) is a harm reduction strategy for People who Inject Drugs (PWIDs) also widely known as opioid substitution therapy (OST), that aims to treat opioid dependence by prescribing methadone to replace illicit opioid narcotics such as heroin. MAT is the use of medications in combination with counseling and behavioral therapies to provide a whole-patient approach to the treatment of substance use disorders. MAT has proven benefits in helping people to reduce illicit opiate use, improving social acceptance and the PWID's health status and reduce criminality (Mattick et al., 2009)

MAT ensures that recovering PWIDs return to a healthier lifestyle, they are able to give back to the community much more than was invested in their MAT treatment. This is very different to PWIDs who are a burden to the community due to their criminal, violent and other anti-social behaviors depleting society resources (Demetrovics et al., 2009) MAT has shown to be effective at improving the survival of PWIDs (Kimber et al., 2010).

The MAT treatment using methadone is a "phased" one, the first step involves intensive stabilization, including withdrawal management, assessment, medication induction, and involvement in psychosocial counseling. The middle phase of care emphasizes medication maintenance and deeper work in and out of counseling on patient goals. In the third phase, "ongoing rehabilitation," the patient and provider might choose to detoxify from all medication or pursue indefinite maintenance, depending on the patient's needs (Moolchan et al., 1994).

Treatment in a phased model, regardless of how long medication is used, involves participation in psychosocial treatment, and engagement with the self-help community. As such, participants in MAT can transition to a lifestyle consistent with being "in recovery" to treat their substance use disorder. All the "phases" of MAT treatment require timely and accurate information, constant and reliable communication between the recovering PWID and healthcare provider and real-time client surveillance during ongoing rehabilitation. Mobile phone technologies can reliably meet this need.

About 6 billion, Over 75% of the world has access to mobile phone subscription (Tomlinson et al., 2013). The World Health Organization (WHO) defines mobile health (mHealth) as "medical and public health practice supported by mobile devices, such as mobile phones, patient monitoring devices, personal digital assistants and other portable wireless devices". mHealth solutions are expected to improve access and outcomes of treatment

(Heerden et al., 2012) with thier use ranging from improving data collection at healthcare service delivery points (Tomlinson et al., 2009) to providing healthcare provider communication to pregnant mothers and their babies as demonstrated in a South African township facing multiple health risks (Rotheram-Borus et al., 2011). Another potential use mobile phone technology is communicating with patients to promote treatment uptake as the pilot in Uganda's Mbarara district showed (Siedner et al., 2012) and the use of mobile phones to monitor treatment adherence in real-time (Haberer et al., 2012).

There is great enthusiasm in the use of mobile phone technologies in provision of public health services to improve access an quality of healthcare. The enthusiasm is driven by both the potential benefits, availability of the technology and level of skills needed to use mobile phones (Leon et al., 2012).

## Mobile Phone Technologies

Short Message Service (SMS) is a standardized communication protocol that allows mobile phone devices exchange short text messages in not more than 160 characters that include alphanumeric and non-text messages (Puneet, 2014). SMSs are in different classes identified by the storage location and importance of the delivered message (Muliticom, 2004; Nokia, 2011), there are four SMS classes. Class 0 SMSs are messages that are displayed on the device screen and a delivery report sent to the sender, this class of message is not saved into the phone memory unless the recipient choose to do so (Nokia, 2011). Class 0 SMSs are also referred to as "Flash SMS" (Ooredoo, 2014).

The use of SMS in public health is on the increase, SMSs are being used to support behavior change and treatment compliance on diabetes management (Cole-Lewis & Kershaw, 2010). SMSs in coded languages to enhance patient privacy have been used as a reminder system to antiretroviral therapy (ART) by sending simple but concise reminder messages (Curioso et al., 2009). There is high acceptability of the use of SMSs in treatment management and adherence (Sahm et al., 2009). It has also been found that SMS have improved appointment attendance by patients (Da Costa et al., 2010). SMSs have also been used to remind patients of their prescription information, this included practical information on drug administration and adverse reaction indications, positive health outcomes and patient satisfaction were realized (Mao et al., 2008).

Unstructured Supplementary Service Data (USSD) is a GSM technology used to send text messages from a mobile phone to a remote server via the

GSM network. The two-way communication of information connection occurs during a "session" when a connection between the two remains open and the process of exchanging messages is ongoing (Viswanathan, 2014; Rouse, 2014). USSD messages support upto 182 alphanumeric characters in length; the process of data exchanges is interactive with the system information exchange guided by a user's inputs (Unstructured Supplementary Service Data, 2014).

There are few documented potential uses of USSD in public health, to meet its need for high notification rate on Tuberculosis (TB) a communicable disease spread by tiny airborne particles Botswana explored the design of a USSD platform to aid tracing close contact of identified patients for testing of the disease (Mosweunyane et al., 2014). In an effort to explore effectiveness of a two-way SMS campaign in HIV prevention in South Africa, a prototype of USSD was developed and used by Female participants to complete a 10-item questionnaire. 68% of the participants were "very interested" in the USSD technology and 62% found it "very Comfortable". This study's findings portrays USSD messaging as an acceptable service to relay health-related messaging (Merrill et al., 2013). There are proposals to use USSD to access treatment guidelines (Littman-Quinn et al., 2012)

Geographical Information Systems (GIS) is the collection of hardware, software geographical data to capture, store, retrieve, analyze and display processed geographical outputs. GIS has made it possible to link public health surveillance data with population demographics, boundaries and nature (Kaushal & Johnson, 2003). Advancement in computing resources to analyze spatial data is providing tools to enhance geographical research on diseases with remote sensing and other GIS platforms serving as enabling technologies in public health (Cromley, 2003). GIS can be applied in cohort identification, disease exposure assessment, mapping of disease incidence and public health surveillance (Jacquez et al., 2005).

## TECHNOLOGY INTEGRATION IN MEDICATION ASSISTED THERAPY

The "phased" MAT treatment using methadone could be enhanced by the integrating mobile technologies including SMS, USSD and mobile GIS for treatment support. The technologies will enable healthcare providers pass relevant messages to recovering PWIDs, avail a system that could be accessed from any location with up-to-date behavior and psychosocial support messages and also provide healthcare providers with an information system that could track defaulters, potentially trace drug overdosed patients or those with special medical needs but are not able to get the health facility.

During the stabilization phase class 0 SMSs sent the recovering PWID or their peer could assist in the identification and management of withdrawal symptoms, relaying of psychosocial support messages to the patient. The class 0 SMS alerts could also serve as a reminder system for daily clinic visits with details of appointment time, treatment buddy contacts and other relevant information. USSD technology could also be used during this phase to avail patients with an accurate interactive platform to access MAT treatment information and support. GIS enabled devices with minimal or no resale value could be provided to patients to make it easier to track and find treatment defaulters or those that may have fallen sick and are unable to get to the health facility. GIS information could also inform a convenient location of a MAT clinic.

The medication maintenance phase of MAT could also benefit from technology integration; SMS alerts could also serve as a reminder system for daily clinic visits, counseling messages and behavior change messages could be relayed to the recovering patients. The USSD technology could still be used as an interactive platform to access MAT treatment information and support. During ongoing rehabilitation, patients could continuously be provided with treatment support by both the SMS and USSD technologies.

## FUTURE RESEARCH DIRECTIONS

USSD is a mobile phone technology that could provide PWIDs with anonymous and confidential platform for PWIDs to access accurate and up-to-date harm reduction information, further research on its potential use and expected positive outcomes should be considered. With the emergence of cheaper, portable and reliable GIS devices, there is need to evaluate their potential benefits to MAT in the tracking, tracing and treatment adherence follow-up for both patients and healthcare providers.

## Conclusion

MAT as a harm reduction strategy for PWIDs in the treat of opioid dependence has potential benefits to the drug user, their family and the community. MAT combined with psychosocial support could reduce drug use, criminal behavior and improve reforming addict's community acceptance and reintegration.

Availability of cheaper, efficient and reliable mobile phones creates technological opportunities to offer secure and confidential access to harm reduction information to PWIDs. Development and customization of mobile phone technology applications to effectively support MAT intervention for PWIDs will increase information access for client literacy, support and monitor MAT treatment and also geographically observe patient trends.

## References

Cole-Lewis, H., & Kershaw, T. (2010). Text messaging as a tool for behavior change in disease prevention and management. *Epidemiologic reviews*, *32*(1), 56-69.

Cromley, E. K. (2003). GIS and disease. *Annual Review of Public Health*,*24*(1), 7-24.

Curioso, W. H., Quistberg, D. A., Cabello, R., Gozzer, E., Garcia, P. J., Holmes, K. K., & Kurth, A. E. (2009). "It's time for your life": How should we remind patients to take medicines using short text messages?. In *AMIA Annual Symposium Proceedings* (Vol. 2009, p. 129). American Medical Informatics Association.

Da Costa, T. M., Salomão, P. L., Martha, A. S., Pisa, I. T., & Sigulem, D. (2010). The impact of short message service text messages sent as appointment reminders to patients' cell phones at outpatient clinics in Sao Paulo, Brazil. *International Journal of Medical Informatics*, *79*(1), 65-70.

Demetrovics, Z., Farkas, J., Csorba, J., Németh, A., Mervó, B., Szemelyácz, J., Fleischmann, E., Kasai-Farkas, A., Petke, Z., Oroján, T., Rózsa, S., Rigó, P., Funk, S., Kapitány, M., Kollár, A., & Rácz, J. (2009).Early experience with Buprenorphine/Naloxonmaintenancetherapy in Hungary. *Neuropsychopharmacol Hung, 11*,249-257. [Online] Available: http:// www.mppt.hu/images/magazin/pdf/xi-evfevfolyam-4-szam/fenntarto-suboxone-terapiaval-szerzett-kezdeti-tapasztalatok.pdf

Eng, T. R., Maxfield, A., Patrick, K., Deering, M. J., Ratzan, S. C., & Gustafson, D. H. (1998). Access to health information and support: a public highway or a private road?. *Jama*, *280*(15), 1371-1375.

Hasanović, M., Pajević, I., Kuldija, A., Delić, A., Sutović, A., & Stanišić, D. (2012). Medical Assisted Treatment of Opiate Dependence with Buprenorphine/Naloxon (Buprenorphine/Naloxon) of Heroin Addicts in Prison who are Aging Penalties. *European Psychiatry, 27*(1). 1-36.

Hasanović,I. M., Kuldija,A., Pajević,M. I., & Zorić, S. (2012).Gender aspects of epidemiological characteristics of heroin addicts clinically treated in psychiatry department from North-Eastern post-war Bosnia and Herzegovina. *Acta Medica Saliniana,41*,17-21.

Jacquez, G. M., Greiling, D. A., & Kaufmann, A. M. (2005). Design and implementation of a space-time intelligence system for disease surveillance. *Journal of Geographical Systems*, *7*(1), 7-23.

Kaushal, A., & Johnson, C. P. (2003, December). Disease Surveillance Using GIS and Remote Sensing. In *Indo-French Workshop.*

Kimber J, et al. *BMJ* 2010;340:c3172

Littman-Quinn, R., Luberti, A. A., & Kovarik, C. (2012). mHealth to Revolutionize Information Retrieval in Low and Middle Income Countries: Introduction and Proposed Solutions Using Botswana as Reference Point. *Studies in health technology and informatics*, *192*, 894-898.

Mao, Y., Zhang, Y., & Zhai, S. (2008). Mobile phone text messaging for pharmaceutical care in a hospital in China. *Journal of telemedicine and Telecare*, *14*(8), 410-414.

Marlatt, G. A., & Witkiewitz, K. (2002). Harm reduction approaches to alcohol use: Health promotion, prevention, and treatment. *Addictive behaviors*, *27*(6), 867-886.

Mattick R, et al. Methadone maintenance therapy versus no opioid replacement therapy for opioid dependence. *Cochrane Database of Systematic Reviews*2009, Issue 3.

Mehić-Basara, N., Oručm, L., Kapur-Pojskić, L., & Ramić, J. (2013).Association of dopamine receptor gene polymorphism and psychological personality traits in liability for opioid addiction. *Bosn J Basic Med Sci.,13*,158-162.

Merrill, J., Hershow, R., Gannett, K., & Barkley, C. (2013, December). Pretesting an mHealth intervention for at-risk adolescent girls in Soweto, South Africa: studying the additive effects of SMSs on improving sexual reproductive health & rights outcomes. In *Proceedings of the Sixth*

*International Conference on Information and Communications Technologies and Development: Notes-Volume 2* (pp. 96-99). ACM.

Moolchan, E.T., & Hoffman, J.A. (1994). Phases of treatment: a practical approach to methadone maintenance treatment [Electronic Version]. *International Journal of the Addictions. 29 (2)*, 135-160.

Mosweunyane, G., Seipone, T., Nkgau, T. Z., & Makhura, O. J. (2014) *Design of A USSD System for TB Contact Tracing.* Retrieved om 1st December 2014 http://www.actapress.com/PaperInfo.aspx?PaperID=456061& reason=500

Muliticom (2004).What is an SMS? Retrieved on 1st December 2014 http://www.gsm-technology.com/gsm.php/en,unlock,subpage_id,smsfaq.html

Nokia (2011). Types of SMS Service Retrieved on 1st December 2014 http://devlib.symbian.slions.net/s3/GUID-CBFDD753-BAE3-5C40-B947-EB8CDA11CD23.html

Ooredoo (2014).Flash SMS Retrieved on 1st December 2014 http://www.nawras.om/personal/talk/extras/messagingcallmanagement/flashsms.aspx

Phillips, G., Felix, L., Galli, L., Patel, V., & Edwards, P. (2010). The effectiveness of M-Health technologies for improving health and health services: a systematic review protocol. *BMC research notes*, *3*(1), 250.

Puneet, G (2014) Short Message Service: What, How and Where? Retrieved on 1st December 2014 http://www.wirelessdevnet.com/channels/sms/features/sms.html

Rekart, M. L. (2006). Sex-work harm reduction. *The Lancet*, *366*(9503), 2123-2134.

Rouse, M (2014) USSD (Unstructured Supplementary Service Data) Retrieved on 1st December 2014 http://searchnetworking.techtarget.com/definition/USSD

Sahm, L., MacCurtain, A., Hayden, J., Roche, C., & Richards, H. L. (2009). Electronic reminders to improve medication adherence—are they acceptable to the patient?. *Pharmacy world & science*, *31*(6), 627-629.

Single, E. (1995). Defining harm reduction. *Drug and alcohol review, 14(3)*, 287-290.

Tamrat, T., & Kachnowski, S. (2012). Special delivery: an analysis of m-Health in maternal and newborn health programs and their outcomes around the world. *Maternal and child health journal*, *16*(5), 1092-1101.

Unit, P. M. S. S. (2004). Alcohol harm reduction strategy for England. *London: Cabinet Office.*

Unstructured Supplementary Service Data (USSD) Retrieved on 1st December 2014 http://www.telecomspace.com/messaging-ussd.html

Viswanathan, P (2014). Definition of USSD Retrieved on 1st December 2014 http://mobiledevices.about.com/od/glossary/g/Definition-Of-Ussd.htm

WHO, UNODC, UNAIDS. (2004). Substitution maintenance therapy in the management of opioid dependence and HIV/AIDS prevention: position paper.

# INDEX

## #

20th century, 64
21st century, 29, 43, 64

## A

abuse, 39, 126
access, vii, xi, 1, 7, 8, 15, 16, 20, 25, 71, 117, 118, 120, 121, 122, 125, 126, 127, 128, 129, 130, 131
active site, 54
adipocytes, viii, 47, 49, 51, 57, 58
adipose tissue, 51
adiposity, ix, 48
administrative support, 18
administrators, 5, 20, 114
adolescent development, 6
adolescents, 15, 28, 30, 32, 71, 81, 84, 90
adrenal glands, 49
adults, 17, 25, 57, 58, 66, 67, 68, 74, 81, 84, 86, 90
advancement, 43
adverse effects, 68, 84
advocacy, 45, 126
aesthetics, 95, 103
Africa, 102, 112, 113, 118
African-American, 43
agencies, 16, 20, 74
aggression, 18
aggressive behavior, 16, 29
agonist, 50, 54, 57
agriculture, 58, 98, 111
AIDS, 117, 120, 125
air quality, 66, 76
airborne particles, 129
alcohol abuse, 22
alcohol consumption, 58
alcohol use, 132
aldosterone, 59
alters, 49
American Psychological Association, 5, 8, 9, 13, 14, 15, 16, 26
Americans with Disabilities Act, 41
anaerobic digesters, 104
androgen, 50, 54, 57, 58
androgens, 49, 54
anemia, 40
anger, 9, 21
ANOVA, 87
antiandrogens, viii, 48
antidepressants, 49
antisocial behavior, 18, 19
anxiety, 31
aromatase inhibitors, ix, 48, 49
arrests, 8
asbestos, 95
Asia, 113, 118
assault, 18
assessment, 19, 20, 21, 22, 28, 30, 31, 127, 129

asthma, ix, x, 66, 67, 74, 77, 83, 84, 85, 86, 87, 88, 89, 90, 91
asthmatic smokers, x, 84
asthmatic symptoms, 89
athletes, 12, 41, 45
atmosphere, 52
atrophy, 40
attacker, 20
attitudes, 24, 72, 78, 106
authorities, viii, 8, 36, 106, 107, 109

## B

bacteria, 49, 100
ban, ix, 63, 65, 66, 67, 70, 72, 74, 76, 77, 78, 105, 108
Bangladesh, 113, 115
barriers, ix, 7, 55, 64, 73
behavioral change, 72, 80
behavioral problems, 14
behaviors, ix, 5, 9, 16, 17, 27, 28, 31, 36, 71, 80, 83, 132
benefits, viii, 36, 58, 66, 101, 127
bias, 73, 96
biodiesel, 98
biosynthesis, 54
biotin, 40
birth rate, 77
birth weight, 97
births, 56
birthweight, 77, 110, 111
bisphenol, 60
Bisphenol A (BPA), viii, 48, 49, 52, 56, 57, 58
blood, 38, 39, 40, 44, 49, 57, 95
blood-brain barrier, 57
bloodstream, 49
body fat, 51
body fluid, 95
body mass index (BMI), 48, 58
Bosnia, 132
Botswana, 129, 132
Brazil, 47, 48, 49, 131
breast cancer, 36, 42, 45, 56
breast milk, 53
breeding, x, 93
bullying, 8, 20, 21, 34
burdensomeness, 22
Bureau of Justice Statistics, 28
businesses, 68, 75, 76
by-products, 52

## C

calcium, 40, 49
caloric intake, 49
Cambodia, 115
campaigns, 14, 38
cancer, 14, 42, 48, 62, 96, 110
capacity building, ix, 64, 73
carbohydrate, 51
carcinogenicity, 56
cardiomyopathy, 40
cardiovascular disease, 44, 48
cardiovascular risk, 57
cardiovascular system, 51
categorization, 6, 96
category a, 99
causal attribution, 85
CDC, 4, 76, 78, 79
cell division, 55
cell phones, 131
cereal fortification, viii, 35
cerebral palsy, 37
challenges, 9, 34, 65, 81, 106, 109, 114, 115
chemical, 50, 52, 55, 56, 58, 95, 96, 98, 100, 101, 110, 121
chemical properties, 52, 98
chemical stability, 58
chemicals, viii, 47, 49, 50, 52, 59, 96, 98
childhood, 27, 37, 38, 56, 67, 77
children, viii, ix, 2, 13, 15, 16, 17, 28, 32, 39, 48, 64, 65, 66, 67, 72, 74, 110
Chile, 63
China, 70, 109, 114, 132
cholesterol, 58
chromosomal abnormalities, 97
cigarette smoking, 70, 80, 84, 90, 91
cities, 98, 103, 115
civil liberties, 9

classes, 53, 57, 128
clients, xi, 125
climates, 18
clinical depression, 22
clinical trials, 42
coal, 103
cognitive dissonance, 85, 88, 89, 90
cognitive theory, 73, 90
college campuses, 29
colon, 48, 96
coma, 40
communication, xi, 17, 25, 70, 89, 105, 125, 127, 128, 129
communication technologies, xi, 125
communities, 2, 13, 15, 25, 34, 40, 44, 66, 67, 68, 69, 70, 72, 73, 74, 101, 103, 104, 106, 118
community, vii, viii, 1, 17, 23, 24, 25, 32, 36, 37, 38, 39, 40, 41, 68, 72, 74, 78, 90, 91, 94, 103, 104, 105, 106, 107, 108, 111, 126, 127, 131
comparative analysis, 30
complexity, 94
compliance, 128
complications, 56, 126
composting, 104, 115
compounds, 53, 54, 55, 56, 58, 59
computing, 129
conception, 38, 40
congenital malformations, 97, 111
conservation, 98
consumption, ix, 16, 59, 63, 64, 66, 69, 71, 88, 98, 103
containers, 99, 101
contaminant, 52
contaminated soil, 105
contamination, 38, 52, 102, 103
contradiction, x, 84, 85
control condition, 70
cooking, 99, 103, 111
cooperation, ix, 64, 73
COPD, 74
coronary heart disease, 80
corticosteroids, 84
cortisol, 59
cosmetics, viii, 48, 52
cost, xi, 21, 29, 100, 102, 107, 108, 117, 119, 120, 121
cotinine, 74
counseling, 21, 42, 78, 127, 130
crimes, 7
criminal behavior, 126, 131
criminality, 127
criminals, 8
crops, 98
cryptorchidism, 55
culture, 19, 95, 107
cure, 85
cystic fibrosis, 39, 40, 45
cytochrome, 59
cytometry, 120
cytoplasm, 50

## D

damages, ix, 63, 64
data collection, 128
database, 45
DDT, viii, 48, 52, 53
deaths, vii, x, 1, 3, 13, 23, 37, 64, 69, 93, 97, 108
decontamination, 100
defects, viii, 35, 36, 37, 40, 97, 110
deficiency, 40, 44, 56, 119
degenerative joint disease, 48
degradation, 50, 56, 59, 99
delinquency, 29
delinquent behavior, 127
demographic characteristics, 67
Department of Education, 4, 8, 10, 11, 16, 18, 23, 28, 29, 34
Department of Homeland Security, 23
Department of Justice, 28
depression, 20, 22
derivatives, 52
desensitization, 16
detection, 45, 120, 121
detergents, 52, 56
developed countries, 70, 71, 75, 100, 102, 104, 108

developing countries, viii, 48, 70, 98, 101, 102, 104, 105, 108, 109, 112
diabetes, 36, 38, 39, 44, 57, 58, 59, 128
diarrhea, 119
diet, 51, 58
dietary habits, 49
dietary prevention, viii, 35
digital cameras, 7
dioxin, 56, 104
dioxine, viii, 48
disability, 36, 37, 40
disclosure, xi, 117, 119
discrimination, xi, 36, 41, 117, 119
diseases, vii, x, 93, 94, 95, 103, 108, 129
disengagement beliefs, ix, x, 83, 84, 85, 87, 88, 89
disinfection, 96, 100, 112
disorder, 7, 127
disposition, 94
dissonance, ix, 83, 85, 88
distribution, 50, 54, 55
District of Columbia, 69
DNA, 38, 39, 44, 50, 54, 55, 57, 58
DNA repair, 57
dopamine, 54, 132
dose-response relationship, ix, 48, 71
Down syndrome, 40
drug abuse, 42
drug use, x, xi, 117, 118, 122, 126, 131
drugs, x, 5, 20, 52, 55, 57, 71, 117, 119, 121, 126
dumping, 97, 101, 102, 106, 108, 115
dyes, 52
dyslipidemia, 48

## E

economic consequences, 70
economic evaluation, 76
economic incentives, 102
economic indicator, 68
economic status, 6, 105
economics, 68
EDCs, viii, 47, 49, 51, 52, 53, 54, 55, 56, 57, 59
education, 94
effluents, 52, 95
embryonic stem cells, 38
emergency, 21, 23, 24, 25, 77, 90
emergency management, 23
emergency preparedness, 23, 25
emergency response, 21
emission, 99
empathy, xi, 117, 119
employees, 107
employers, 70
employment, 41, 68
empowerment, 105
encephalopathy, 40
endocrine, viii, 48, 49, 50, 51, 52, 54, 55, 57, 59, 60, 62
endocrine disorders, 55
endocrine function, viii, 48, 49
endocrine glands, 49
endocrine system, 49, 50, 51, 52, 55
endocrine-disrupting chemicals, 49
endocrinology, 60
endometriosis, 56
energy, 39, 48, 50, 51, 57, 62
enforcement, 103
England, 67, 109, 133
environment, viii, x, 15, 36, 38, 44, 49, 52, 55, 57, 75, 91, 94, 100, 101, 104, 105, 108
environmental change, 70
environmental contaminants, viii, ix, 35, 48, 51
environmental contamination, 111
environmental movement, 103
environmental policy, 112
environmental protection, 104
Environmental Protection Agency (EPA), 61
environmental regulations, 98
environmental standards, 102, 103
environmental variables, 14
environmentalism, 104
environments, 18, 38
enzymes, 40, 51, 54, 59
epidemic, ix, 60, 63, 64, 65, 75, 108

epidemiologic, 61, 110
epidemiologic studies, 61
epidemiology, 45, 112
epigenetic mechanisms, viii, 36
epigenetics, 36
epispadias, 97
equipment, 120, 121
estrogen, 49, 50, 51, 54, 55, 56, 57, 58
ethics, 43
ethnic background, 19
ethnic groups, 38, 43
etiology, 59
eugenics, 40, 42
Europe, 101, 103, 111, 118
evacuation, 25
evidence, ix, xi, 2, 7, 8, 10, 11, 16, 22, 23, 27, 42, 43, 45, 46, 55, 59, 63, 64, 65, 66, 68, 69, 70, 71, 72, 73, 74, 75, 79, 80, 117
evil, 12
expenditures, 69
experimental condition, 70
exports, 105
exposure, viii, ix, 11, 16, 35, 36, 38, 44, 48, 49, 51, 52, 54, 56, 57, 58, 59, 60, 64, 66, 71, 74, 77, 81, 96, 98, 129
expulsion, 5, 33
extrinsic motivation, 80

## F

false positive, 9
family history, 42, 45, 46
family members, 15
family system, 37
fat, ix, 48, 49, 50, 51, 57, 58
fatty acids, 50, 99
FCTC, ix, 63, 64, 65, 72, 73, 75
Federal Bureau of Investigation (FBI), 8, 9, 10, 17, 20, 21, 26, 33
feelings, 19, 21
fetal growth, 38
fetus, 37, 38, 53, 55, 57
financial resources, 106
financial support, 107
Finland, 67
firearms, 3, 5, 7, 8, 15, 19, 20, 26, 30
fish, 59
flame retardants, 56
flexibility, xi, 117, 119
fluctuations, 55
folate, 37
folic acid, 37
food, viii, 35, 37, 38, 48, 53, 57, 59, 95, 98
food chain, 59
food production, 98
force, 106, 109
foundations, 29, 90
Framework Convention on Tobacco Control, ix, 63, 64, 65, 75
fraud, 101
funding, 16, 120

## G

garbage, 98
gastroschisis, 97
gene expression, 38, 42, 45, 58
gene-environment interactions, viii, 36
genes, 37, 38, 39, 44, 50, 55
genetic mutations, 55
genetic predisposition, 37, 48
genetic programs, 37
genetic screening, 41
genetic testing, viii, 35, 36
genetics, viii, 35, 37, 42, 43, 44, 91
genomics, 45, 46
Germany, 4, 40, 81
gestational diabetes, 38
GIS, 129, 130, 131, 132
global scale, 101
glucocorticoid, 57
glucocorticoids, 50
glucose, 38, 39, 51, 57
gonads, 49
governments, 102, 104
Greece, 41
gross national product, 102
groundwater, 52, 102
growth, x, 50, 51, 54, 57, 93
growth hormone, 51, 54, 57

Guatemala, 113
guidelines, 21, 27, 59, 119, 121, 129
Guinea, 102
gun violence, vii, 1, 13, 15, 16, 26, 32

## H

Haiti, 102
harm reduction, vii, x, xi, 35, 93, 109, 118, 119, 125, 126, 127, 130, 131, 133
harmful effects, 16, 89, 126
hazardous waste, 95, 96, 97, 101, 102, 105, 108, 110, 111
hazardous wastes, 101, 102, 105, 108
hazards, 36, 100, 102, 109
health, vii, ix, x, xi, 14, 24, 35, 36, 37, 38, 39, 41, 42, 43, 44, 45, 49, 52, 60, 62, 63, 64, 65, 66, 67, 69, 70, 71, 72, 74, 75, 76, 80, 81, 84, 86, 88, 89, 90, 93, 94, 96, 100, 108, 111, 113, 117, 119, 122, 125, 126, 127, 128, 129, 130, 132, 133
health care, xi, 37, 69, 75, 117, 119
health care costs, 69, 75
health condition, 14
health effects, 49, 62
health information, 132
health insurance, 41
health practitioners, 41
health problems, 96
health promotion, ix, 63, 64, 65
health risks, 71, 72, 128
health services, 133
health status, 127
health system, vii, 94
hearing loss, 40
heart attack, 67
heart disease, 71
heavy metals, 52, 55
helplessness, 19
hemoglobinopathies, 36, 39, 40
hemorrhage, 56
hepatitis, 126
hepatosplenomegaly, 40
heroin, 118, 119, 126, 127, 132
heroin addicts, 132
heterozygote, 40, 45
high blood pressure, 36
HIV/AIDS, x, 117, 118, 119, 121, 122, 126, 129, 134
homeostasis, viii, 39, 47, 49, 52, 54, 57, 59
homicide, vii, 1, 3, 13, 19, 21, 32
hopelessness, 22
hormone, 50, 51, 54, 55, 56
hormones, viii, 47, 49, 50, 51, 52, 54, 55, 56, 59
hospitality, 66, 68, 74, 76, 77, 78, 81
hospitalization, 21
human behavior, 56
human body, 52, 59
human capital, ix, 64, 73
human health, 56, 105
human resources, 120, 121
human right, 105, 108
Hungary, 131
hyperinsulinemia, 58
hypertension, 48
hypospadias, 55, 97
hypothalamus, 56, 57
hypothyroidism, 57
hypoxia, 37

## I

identification, 100, 129, 130
ideology, 105
immediate situation, 21
immune system, 57
immunization, 96
Impact Assessment, 112
imprinting, 39
improvements, 24, 27, 67, 73, 84
incidence, 37, 55, 59, 67, 96, 97, 110, 129
income, viii, 35, 74, 106, 113, 114
incompatibility, 88
independent variable, x, 83
India, 114
individuals, 2, 3, 8, 11, 13, 17, 19, 22, 41, 42, 58, 59, 73, 84, 86, 89, 94
induction, 38, 127
industrial chemicals, 59

industrial revolution, 98, 103, 108
industrial wastes, 98
industrialization, 101
industrialized countries, 101, 102, 103
industry, 52, 58, 68, 74, 75, 77, 78
ineffectiveness, 104
inequality, 101
infant mortality, 97
infection, 94, 99, 112, 118
infertility, 55
informal sector, 106, 107
Information and Communication Technologies, 126
information exchange, 129
infrastructure, 24, 103, 106, 112, 120, 121
inheritance, 38
initiation, 80, 119, 120, 122
injuries, 13, 21, 25, 36, 42, 119
insomnia, 22
institutions, 16, 104
insulin, 51, 57, 58
insulin resistance, 57, 58
integration, 130
intelligence, 132
interference, viii, 47, 49
international standards, 99
intervention, vii, xi, 2, 14, 20, 21, 23, 24, 26, 27, 28, 29, 31, 32, 33, 70, 72, 73, 108, 125, 126, 131, 132
intervention strategies, 14
intrauterine development, viii, 47, 57, 58
investment, 103, 106
iodine, 56
ionizing radiation, 100
Iran, 114
Ireland, 67, 68, 69, 78
isoflavone, 57
isolation, 10, 41
Israel, 83, 115
Italy, 67, 69, 76, 78, 101

J

Jordan, 115
juvenile crime, 13

K

Kenya, x, xi, 117, 118, 119, 125

L

labeling, viii, 9, 10, 36, 41, 42
lactose-free formula, 40
landfills, 52, 100, 104, 106, 115
Latin America, 113
law enforcement, vii, 1, 3, 8, 11, 20, 21, 24, 25
laws, 4, 5, 20, 66, 67, 68, 69, 70, 74, 75, 76, 77, 78, 79, 102
leaching, 97, 104
lead, viii, 3, 16, 25, 35, 36, 38, 39, 44, 54, 56, 58, 69, 75
leakage, 10, 20
leaks, 98
legality, 6
legislation, 5, 66, 67, 68, 73, 74, 75, 76, 77, 78, 81, 103, 106, 108
leptin, 39, 51
level of education, 106
life expectancy, 40
limb weakness, 40
lipid metabolism, 51, 57
lipogenesis, ix, 48, 49, 50, 58
lipolysis, 50
literacy, xi, 41, 45, 125, 126, 131
liver, 40, 48, 51, 57, 96
liver enzymes, 57
local authorities, 103, 105, 107
localization, 96
Love Canal, 96, 97, 110
low birthweight, 110, 111
lubricants, 52
lung cancer, 14, 71
lung function, 84

M

management, 21, 28, 30, 33, 60, 67, 94, 99, 100, 103, 104, 105, 106, 107, 108, 109,

112, 113, 114, 115, 120, 122, 127, 128, 130, 131, 134
manure, 95, 98
mapping, 129
mass, viii, 16, 48, 50, 57
mastectomy, 42
materials, 12, 95, 98, 107, 119
maternal smoking, 68, 70, 79
matter, 40, 105, 106, 108
media, vii, 1, 2, 8, 10, 12, 13, 16, 69
medical, 24, 37, 45, 59, 60, 127, 130
medication, 67, 89, 126, 127, 130, 133
medicine, 43, 45
mellitus, 48
memory, 40, 56, 128
mental health, 21, 22, 23, 24, 25, 28
mental health professionals, 22, 23, 24, 25
mental retardation, 37, 40, 57
MES, 60
meta-analysis, 67, 77
metabolic defects, viii, 35
metabolic disorder, 49, 51
metabolic disorders, 49, 51
metabolic syndrome, 58
metabolism, viii, 36, 39, 40, 44, 47, 51, 52, 54, 55
metabolites, 40
metals, 95, 98
methadone, 127, 129, 133
methyl groups, 38
methylation, 38, 39, 44, 55, 58
Middle East, 11, 30
migration, 98
mild asthma, 90
mineralocorticoid, 50
Minneapolis, 67
minorities, 74
minority groups, 36
miscarriages, 56
misunderstanding, 2
mobile device, 127
mobile phone, xi, 125, 126, 127, 128, 130, 131
models, vii, 14, 20, 35, 113
modernisation, 114
mood change, 17
morbidity, 48
mortality, ix, 37, 42, 44, 48, 59, 63, 64, 69, 79, 84, 110
mortality rate, 69
mortality risk, 42
motivation, 11, 22, 69, 71, 72, 107, 114
municipal solid waste, 110, 112, 113, 115
murder, vii, 1, 2, 11, 12, 13, 16, 22, 30
murder-suicide, vii, 1
musculoskeletal, 98
musculoskeletal system, 98
mutations, 45
myocardial infarction, ix, 64, 65, 66, 77

## N

Namibia, 102
narcotics, 126, 127
National Center for Education Statistics, 28
natural disasters, 24
natural resources, 98
negative consequences, 126
negative effects, 16
negative outcomes, 7, 16
Nepal, 114
nervous system, ix, 48, 49, 98
Netherlands, 113, 114
networking, 105
neural tube defects, viii, 35, 36, 97
neurons, 57
neurotransmitters, 54, 55
New Zealand, 69
next generation, 40
NGOs, 104, 108
NHS, 75
nicotine, 70, 74
Nigeria, 101, 102, 115
nightmares, 22
NIJ, 32
No Child Left Behind, 6
non-Hodgkin's lymphoma, 96
non-smokers, 74, 85, 88, 89
norepinephrine, 54
North America, 96, 118

NRT, 64, 69
nuclear receptors, ix, 48, 49, 50, 58
nutrition, 58, 60

## O

obesity, viii, 44, 47, 48, 49, 50, 51, 57, 58, 59, 60, 61
oesophageal, 96
Office of Justice Programs, 28
oil, 99, 111
Oklahoma, 13
olanzapine, 57
omission, vii, 35, 36
operating costs, 66
opportunities, xi, 70, 125, 126, 131
organ, 56, 94, 96
organism, 49, 94
organochlorine pesticides, viii, 48
organs, 49, 95
ovarian cancer, viii, 35, 42, 45
ovaries, 51
overnutrition, 39

## P

pancreas, 96
parents, vii, 1, 3, 15, 16, 20, 22, 30, 41
participants, ix, 70, 71, 72, 83, 86, 89, 127, 129
pathogenesis, 49
pathogens, 95
pathways, 54
PCBs, 53, 55, 56, 59
peer group, 20
peer influence, 106
peptic ulcer, 36
per capita income, 110
perceived control, 87
perchlorate, 56
perinatal, 43, 51
perpetrators, vii, 1, 3, 10, 11, 12, 16, 22
persistent asthma, 84
Persistent Organic Pollutants (POPs), 52, 58, 61
personal identity, 42
personality, 94, 132
personality traits, 132
PGD, 40
pharmaceutical, 96, 132
pharmacological treatment, 70
Philadelphia, 43
phthalates, viii, 48, 52, 58
physical health, 24
physiology, 49
phytoestrogens, viii, 48, 52, 55
placenta, 37, 38, 53, 56
placenta previa, 37
plastics, 52, 56, 58, 95, 98
platform, 108, 129, 130
plausibility, 71
police, 7, 25, 118, 119
policy, vii, ix, 1, 3, 15, 26, 36, 41, 45, 64, 65, 70, 77, 78, 79, 80, 103, 104, 121
policy initiative, 15
policymakers, vii, 1, 3, 74, 103
pollutants, 52
pollution, 66, 74, 75, 76, 78, 96, 97, 98, 110, 111
polychlorinated biphenyl, 55, 58, 101, 105
polychlorinated biphenyls (PCBs), 58
polymorphism, 132
population, ix, x, xi, 4, 14, 37, 42, 43, 45, 59, 63, 64, 66, 67, 69, 75, 80, 90, 93, 94, 103, 108, 118, 125, 129
population growth, 94, 108
Portugal, 67
positive interactions, 18
postnatal exposure, viii, 48
potential benefits, 128, 130, 131
poverty, 102
PPARy receptors, viii, 48
pregnancy, 38, 49, 55, 56, 70, 79, 111
prematurity, 110
prenatal genetic testing, viii, 36
preparedness, 24
preservation, 112
prevalence rate, 118

prevention, viii, 10, 14, 15, 16, 18, 22, 23, 24, 26, 27, 28, 29, 30, 31, 32, 34, 35, 36, 37, 38, 39, 40, 42, 43, 44, 45, 59, 70, 73, 98, 111, 118, 119, 129, 131, 132, 134
principles, vii, ix, 6, 22, 54, 63, 65, 105
prisons, 74
private sector, 69, 104, 107, 108
probability, 17, 68, 75
professionalism, 107
professionals, 23
progesterone, 49, 50, 55, 56
programming, 38, 62
prolactin, 54
prolapse, 37
prophylactic, 42
prosocial behavior, 7, 34
prostate cancer, 56
protection, 104, 105
protective factors, 14
proteins, 38, 54, 58
prototype, 129
psychiatry, 132
psychological problems, 96
psychologist, 22, 24
psychology, 33
psychosocial support, 119, 126, 130, 131
public concern, 102
public health, vii, viii, 1, 13, 14, 25, 26, 29, 32, 35, 36, 37, 38, 39, 42, 43, 44, 45, 46, 48, 73, 79, 91, 94, 96, 99, 102, 103, 105, 108, 126, 127, 128, 129
public health genetics, viii, 35, 37
public safety, 100
public schools, 26

## Q

quality control, 121
quality of life, x, 40, 93, 94

## R

race, ix, 44, 63, 65, 105
racism, 101, 105
radioactive waste, 101
radius, 97, 101
ratification, 105
reactions, 50
reagents, 121
real estate, 106
receptors, viii, 48, 49, 50, 51, 54, 55, 56, 57, 58
recognition, 50, 105, 107, 109
recommendations, ix, 23, 26, 63, 65
recovery, 85, 106, 127
recycling, 98, 106, 108, 114
reduction, 118
reform, 112
regulations, 66, 77, 78, 108, 109
regulatory agencies, 59
rehabilitation, 127, 130
religion, ix, 16, 43, 63, 65
remote sensing, 129
renewable energy, 112
reproduction, 43, 50, 52, 97
reserves, 51
residues, 95
resources, viii, 36, 37, 39, 41, 98, 103, 104, 107, 127, 129
response, vii, 2, 11, 21, 23, 24, 25, 26, 28, 29, 50, 59, 84, 97, 119, 120, 121
restaurants, 66, 67, 68, 73, 76, 77, 78
restrictions, 16, 66, 76
retail, 68, 75
retaliation, 17
retardation, 57
rights, 36, 41, 132
risk, vii, x, 2, 5, 9, 14, 15, 16, 18, 19, 20, 22, 24, 25, 29, 30, 32, 33, 38, 39, 41, 42, 56, 58, 59, 68, 71, 73, 77, 80, 84, 85, 93, 96, 97, 111, 118, 126, 132
risk assessment, vii, 2, 19, 22, 29, 59
risk factors, 5, 9, 14, 15, 22, 58, 80
risks, 41, 44, 71, 74, 80, 97
RNA, 38, 120
rural areas, 52

## S

safety, 2, 4, 6, 15, 18, 20, 24, 25, 26, 27, 28, 29, 30, 31, 32, 33, 34, 43, 59, 94, 101, 102, 103, 105
salts, 49
SAMHSA, 21, 33
sanctions, 5, 70
savings, 69, 75
scholarship, 23
school, vii, ix, 1, 2, 3, 4, 5, 6, 7, 8, 9, 10, 11, 12, 13, 14, 16, 17, 18, 19, 20, 21, 22, 23, 24, 25, 26, 27, 28, 29, 30, 31, 32, 33, 34, 64, 65, 70, 72, 73
school climate, 8, 18, 21, 29
school personnel, vii, 1, 3, 7, 17, 20, 21, 22, 23, 24, 25, 30
school shootings, vii, 1, 2, 3, 4, 7, 8, 9, 10, 11, 13, 14, 16, 17, 20, 23, 24, 25, 26, 27, 28, 32, 34
school success, 34
secondary schools, 90
Secret Service, 4, 8, 10, 11, 16, 17, 18, 20, 21, 29, 32, 34
secretion, 52
security, 5, 7, 8, 24, 26, 33, 34
security guard, 7, 8
sedentary lifestyle, 49
sediments, 52
segregation, 99
self-regulation, 51
semen, 55
serotonin, 54, 57
services, viii, xi, 23, 25, 28, 36, 38, 44, 74, 106, 107, 117, 119, 128
settlements, 103
sex, 36, 54, 55
sex hormones, 54
sex steroid, 55
showing, 66
sickle cell, 37, 39, 41, 42, 45
sickle cell anemia, 39
Sierra Leone, 102
signs, 5, 9, 19, 20, 22, 26, 100
simulation, 67, 79
skilled personnel, 107
skin, 53, 96, 119
skin diseases, 119
sleep apnea, 48
sleep deprivation, 49
smoke exposure, 76
smoking, ix, x, 58, 63, 64, 65, 66, 68, 69, 70, 71, 72, 73, 74, 75, 76, 77, 78, 79, 80, 81, 83, 84, 85, 86, 87, 88, 89, 90, 91
smoking ban, ix, 63, 65, 66, 70, 76, 77, 78
smoking cessation, 69, 70, 73, 74, 78, 80, 84, 90
SMS, 128, 129, 130, 133
social acceptance, 127
social behavior, 127
social condition, ix, 63, 65
social environment, 41
social influences, 106
social network, 86
social status, 107
social support, 70, 72
social withdrawal, 22
society, vii, 29, 35, 94, 127
socioeconomic status, 19
software, 129
solid waste, 109, 113, 114, 115
solubility, 52
solution, 105, 107
solvents, 52, 55, 98
South Africa, 115, 128, 129, 132
space-time, 132
Spain, 74
special education, 6
species, 11, 52
spending, 20
sperm, 55
spontaneous abortion, 97
Sri Lanka, 115
stability, 37, 52
stabilization, 54, 127, 130
staff members, 18
stakeholders, 108, 115
state, 6, 9, 37, 43, 55, 67, 68, 69, 79, 85, 100
steroids, 50, 51, 59
storage, 50, 51, 99, 100, 106, 128

stress, 36, 58, 96
sub-Saharan Africa, 118
substance abuse, 36
substance use, 127
Sudden Infant Death Syndrome (SIDS), 67, 77
suicidal behavior, 19, 22, 31, 32
suicidal ideation, 11, 22
suicidal youth, vii, 2
suicide, vii, 1, 10, 11, 12, 13, 15, 19, 22, 26, 29, 30, 32, 33
suicide attempts, 22
suicide bombers, 11, 30
support services, 23
support staff, 24
suppression, 119, 120, 121, 122
surveillance, 7, 8, 33, 38, 127, 129, 132
survival, 38, 127
susceptibility, 51
suspensions, 6, 18, 21, 27
Switzerland, 113
sympathetic nervous system, 51
symptoms, x, 67, 84, 85, 87, 89, 96
synthesis, ix, 48, 49, 50, 52, 54, 55, 59

## T

Taiwan, 79, 98, 111
tamoxifen, 42
target, 4, 5, 7, 10, 12, 14, 18, 50, 54, 57, 58, 74, 108
Task Force, 5, 26
tax data, 68
tax increase, 70, 79
taxes, ix, 64, 65, 69, 75, 79
teachers, 5, 24, 70
teams, 21, 23, 24, 25
techniques, ix, 73, 83
technologies, 42, 107, 127, 128, 129, 133
technology, 40, 43, 44, 100, 126, 128, 129, 130, 131, 132, 133
teratogen, 38
testicular cancer, 55
testing, viii, xi, 36, 40, 41, 42, 96, 118, 120, 121, 122, 129
testosterone, 49, 51, 54, 55
text messaging, 132
textiles, 95
thalassemia, 39
therapy, 40, 120, 126, 127, 128, 132, 134
thiazolidinediones, 57
thoughts, 16, 22, 27, 28, 85
threat assessment, 10, 18, 19, 20, 21, 22, 24, 25, 27, 30, 33
threatening behavior, 19
threats, 5, 17, 20, 21, 27, 32, 64
thyroid, 49, 50, 51, 54, 56, 57
thyroid gland, 56
thyroxin, 49
tibia, 38
time frame, 6
tissue, 50, 54, 58, 59
tobacco, vii, ix, 63, 64, 65, 68, 69, 70, 71, 74, 75, 76, 78, 79, 80, 81
tobacco cessation program, ix, 64, 65
tobacco control, ix, 63, 64, 65
tobacco smoke, 74, 76, 78
tobacco smoking, ix, 63, 65
toxic waste, x, 93, 101, 102, 105, 108, 110
toxicity, 52, 109
training, 21, 24, 25, 30, 68, 107, 109
transcription, 51
transcription factors, 51
transmission, 40, 94, 118, 119
transparency, 105
transplantation, 40
transport, 52, 55, 66
transportation, 54, 73, 99, 100, 105, 106
trauma, 13, 24
treatment, xi, 42, 51, 59, 84, 90, 96, 98, 99, 100, 106, 117, 118, 119, 120, 121, 126, 127, 128, 129, 130, 131, 132, 133
treatment methods, 100
trial, 31
tricyclic antidepressant, 57
tricyclic antidepressants, 57
triiodothyronine, 54
tumor, 42, 45
turnover, 68, 78
type 2 diabetes, 48

## U

Ukraine, 79
umbilical cord, 37
UNDP, 113
United Kingdom (UK), 40, 78, 95, 97, 112, 114
United Nations (UN), ix, 63, 65, 114
United States (USA), viii, 2, 3, 30, 34, 36, 38, 42, 58, 69, 79, 80, 112
universities, 2, 25, 66
urban, x, 68, 93, 104, 114
urban population, 104
urbanization, 94
urine, 58
uterus, 51

## V

vandalism, 18
vector, 94
vegetables, 95
vehicles, 106
vessels, 101
victimization, 32
victims, vii, 1, 11, 25
video games, 9, 16
videos, 12
violence, vii, 1, 3, 4, 6, 7, 8, 10, 11, 13, 14, 15, 16, 17, 18, 20, 23, 26, 27, 28, 29, 30, 31, 32, 33, 34
violent behavior, 5, 9, 14, 15
violent crime, 6
violent entertainment, 16
viruses, 49
vitamin D, 50

## W

Wales, 109
war, 29, 132
Washington, 26, 28, 29, 34, 43, 61, 109
waste, vii, viii, x, 48, 52, 93, 94, 95, 97, 98, 99, 100, 101, 102, 103, 104, 105, 106, 107, 108, 109, 110, 111, 112, 113, 114, 115
waste disposal, 99, 100, 102, 106, 107, 109, 114
waste management, vii, x, 94, 99, 100, 103, 104, 105, 106, 107, 108, 109, 110, 112, 113, 114, 115
waste treatment, 98, 99, 106, 107
water, 52, 53, 102, 103, 110, 112
weapons, 3, 20
weight gain, 38, 40, 51, 57, 58
wellness, 28
wireless devices, 127
withdrawal, 127, 130
withdrawal symptoms, 130
workers, 66, 69, 74, 76, 81, 101, 107, 109
workforce, viii, 36, 70
workplace, 23, 36, 38, 41, 69, 70, 77, 78
World Health Organization (WHO), ix, xi, 48, 60, 61, 63, 64, 65, 66, 75, 117, 118, 119, 126, 127, 134

## Y

young adults, 78
young people, vii, 1, 15, 25, 72, 80, 81

## Z

zinc, 50